ALWAYS ON

Praise for *Always On*

'A brilliant summation of the years that have seen the world transformed in ways that no one predicted and whose effects we are still trying to comprehend – all told from the point of view of someone who was himself *Always On* … This delightfully insightful and intensely readable history combines the personal with the objective. From Jobs to Musk, from Facebook to fake news, from Snapchat to Bitcoin by way of Raspberries, Blackberries and Apples there is an energy and drama to Rory's writing which nonetheless leaves space for us, the reader, to make up our minds just how much of the story he tells is triumph and how much disaster … A superb reminder of how far we have come'

Stephen Fry

'Cellan-Jones weaves together the broad story of the smartphone era with the personal element. By showing how technology has touched – and altered – him for good and bad he shows how it has affected us all'

Jimmy Wales, founder of Wikipedia

'Who better to tell us this story than the arch technology storyteller himself? From the first smartphone to test and trace, Rory has seen it all and interviewed everyone. Putting it all together makes for a fascinating and beautifully written story of our times'

Wendy Hall, Regius Professor of Computer Science, University of Southampton

ALWAYS ON

Hope and Fear in the Social Smartphone Era

RORY CELLAN-JONES

BLOOMSBURY CONTINUUM
LONDON · OXFORD · NEW YORK · NEW DELHI · SYDNEY

BLOOMSBURY CONTINUUM
Bloomsbury Publishing Plc
50 Bedford Square, London, WC1B 3DP, UK
29 Earlsfort Terrace, Dublin 2, Ireland

BLOOMSBURY, BLOOMSBURY CONTINUUM and the Diana logo are trademarks of
Bloomsbury Publishing Plc

First published in Great Britain 2021

A catalogue record for this book is available from the British Library

Library of Congress Cataloguing-in-Publication data has been applied for

ISBN: HB: 978-1-4729-8119-6; TPB: 978-1-4729-9227-7; eBook: 978-1-4729-8117-2;
ePDF: 978-1-4729-8118-9

2 4 6 8 10 9 7 5 3 1

Typeset by Deanta Global Publishing Services, Chennai, India
Printed and bound in Great Britain by CPI Group (UK) Ltd, Croydon CR0 4YY

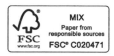

To find out more about our authors and books visit www.bloomsbury.com
and sign up for our newsletters

CONTENTS

PROLOGUE

It is late May in 2019. On the bedside table my phone pings before 6 a.m. My first action, as ever, is to check Twitter to see what has happened in the world since I last looked at midnight before falling asleep. I tumble out of bed, make a cup of tea for my wife and leave the house with the dog. Our collie cross, acquired from a rescue home a dozen years earlier, does need three walks a day, but I am also mindful of the daily exercise target my phone and the smartwatch linked to it have set for me.

In the park, I snap a photo with my phone of Cabbage – yes, that is the name of our pet. As we walk back I post it on Instagram, and an automated piece of software called If This Then That reposts it on Twitter and Facebook. The caption reads, 'An early start on 5G day'.

Checking on the National Rail app that my train is on time, I leave my West London home for what promises to be a landmark day for the device that has transformed the way we live over the past decade. The smartphone.

By around 7.30 I am hurrying along the Strand, conscious that I could be about to make a little piece of technology history. I round a corner and there, parked just yards from Covent Garden's market hall, is an unusually substantial BBC News team.

These days a live news broadcast is an efficient affair. Often there will be a satellite truck with a camera operator, but more frequently there's just one person with a box of tricks that uses a number of mobile phone simcards to connect the reporter to the studio back at base. But today there are actually two vans, two camera operators, a couple of producers, a gaggle of broadcast engineers – plus two worried-looking public relations executives from the mobile phone network EE.

All eyes are on a white cylinder perched on the roof of one of the BBC vans with the word HUAWEI on it. It is a 5G router, and the plan is that this piece of kit will link us up to the *BBC Breakfast* studio in Salford and allow me to tell the audience about an important day for the future of UK technology.

Early this morning EE, the mobile phone company owned by BT, has switched on the first 5G network to serve UK customers. Just a handful of people in a few cities will have the phones needed to access this network, but there is nevertheless a sense of excitement that for once Britain is not being left in the slow lane.

Back in 2000, as a BBC business correspondent, I had covered the extraordinary auction which saw the likes of Vodafone, BT's Cellnet and Orange compete to acquire the 3G spectrum. I watched in the Canary Wharf offices where the auction was run as ever more eye-watering bids arrived on a fax machine. It was the height of the dot.com bubble, when excitement about the potential of the internet and mobile communications persuaded previously sober telecoms executives to throw money at anything which might give them an edge.

In the end, the winners paid an extraordinary £22.5 billion to the Treasury for their 3G licences. Then, as the dot.com bubble burst, they proceeded to do very little; 3G, which promised the dawn of the mobile data era with video calls and all sorts of smart new applications, was slow to arrive in the UK, as if, having spent all that money, the telecoms executives felt the need to sober up again.

When 4G came along, there was even greater caution, and the UK, along with the rest of Europe, fell behind the US and China in rolling out the faster new networks.

But now, in May 2019, the bubble mentality of 20 years ago is back. The predictions that fuelled the first boom – that the internet would transform every aspect of our economy and society – have proved correct, and a few giant organizations have become immensely wealthy and powerful.

Amazon has changed the way we shop, Facebook and Twitter have redefined how we communicate with friends and hear the news, 'to google' has become a verb defining how we understand just about everything.

But above all Apple, with its iPhone which launched the smartphone era, has put vast computing power into the pockets of billions of people. The combination of these extraordinary devices with social networks that have become essential channels of communication at home and at work means we are now in a new age: the social smartphone era.

And, outside China, all the most dominant forces in this new economic paradigm are American. European firms have been mostly passive bystanders, with the pioneering Finnish giant Nokia, the market leader in mobile phones in 2007, irrelevant just five years later.

As for the UK, our great hope for a world-beating tech business, the mobile chip designer Arm, has been snapped up by Japan's SoftBank. Meanwhile, our broadband networks are slow and mobile phone coverage in rural areas is patchy. So as the 5G age dawns in the UK, the mantra from both government and business is – MUST DO BETTER!

There has been a huge amount of hype about what 5G will offer, not just in terms of speed but in the way it will bring about a truly networked economy. The promise is that not just people but every object imaginable – cars, lamp posts, dustbins, every item in a grocery or clothes shop – will be hooked up to the network.

The result will be a transformation of the way our economy and our cities work. Driverless cars will navigate the streets, updated every millisecond on the hazards around them. Thanks to the low latency of the 5G network – in other words, the much shorter delay between pressing a button and seeing an effect – surgeons will be able to conduct remote operations: the moment the human doctor moves, so does the robot medic hundreds of miles away. Sensors across a city's water and sewerage system will give council engineers instant information about burst water mains or flood threats.

That, at least, is the promise, and governments around the world are being told that they need to make 5G happen as quickly as possible, by auctioning off the necessary airwaves and cutting the bureaucracy which might hamper the roll-out.

So in London this May morning there is some satisfaction that, just weeks after South Korea and the United States have launched their first 5G networks, the UK is following suit. True, there has been something of a political hand grenade thrown into the process by the United States. The Trump administration has been warning its allies for months that China's Huawei is a security threat, and should not be allowed anywhere near the 5G networks that are going to be such a critical part of any country's infrastructure.

Over the past 30 years Huawei has grown into the world's leading maker of telecoms equipment, and in under a decade it has come from nowhere to pass Apple as the second biggest seller of smartphones, with the market leader, South Korea's Samsung, in its sights. These days it provides all the kit essential to the roll-out of a new network, from routers to radio equipment, and often at a keener price than its only two rivals, Sweden's Ericsson and Finland's Nokia.

But its rise has been accompanied by suspicions of industrial espionage, and by the fear that a Chinese company will always owe its allegiance to the Communist Party above the security of its customers.

These concerns have been voiced right across the West, but it is the United States which has brought matters to a head. One ally, Australia, has already agreed to bar the Chinese firm from its 5G networks, and pressure is mounting on the government of Theresa May to follow suit. But here's the problem: Huawei kit is all over the UK's existing phone networks. A few days earlier, I had climbed onto a roof in the City of London to watch engineers from EE installing one of the first 5G masts. What that meant in practice was hooking up a piece of Huawei kit to an existing 4G mast that was itself dependent on other equipment from the Chinese company.

All of the big four UK mobile phone companies are planning to start rolling out 5G networks, and three out of four have put Huawei equipment at the heart of their plans. If they are not allowed to use its equipment, they warn, there could be a delay of up to two years in the large-scale deployment of 5G in the UK. Privately, they admit to some concerns about the security of the Chinese company, but they point out that a division of GCHQ has been running a unit examining Huawei's equipment for the past few years. While the signals agency has raised concerns about software security, it has given the mobile firms a cautious nod to use Huawei's gear, as long as they keep it out of the core of their networks.

It is believed the same message has been given to Theresa May's cabinet but, while an announcement of the conclusion of a review had been expected in April, by late May the government has said nothing – and the Trump administration continues to issue dire warnings about the consequences of playing with the Chinese. Do you want to be shut out of the vital Five Eyes intelligence-sharing arrangement? comes the message from the most extreme voices in Washington, and, do you really expect us to sign a post-Brexit trade deal with a supposed ally who is busy cosying up to our great enemy, China?

Immersed in seemingly intractable negotiations about its departure from the EU, the UK government worries and dithers, continuing to put off the decision that is vital to the 5G plans of the mobile firms.

What to do? EE decides to grit its teeth and go ahead with the launch. Which is why I and an anxious BBC team are staring at that Huawei router on the van roof. Several BBC engineers have been testing the equipment in the surrounding streets over the preceding days, and all seems well.

But now we are preparing for a moment in history – the first live television broadcast in Europe over 5G. (We haven't checked, but it seems possible that the South Koreans have already done it.)

I plug in my earpiece, the camera operator Emma clips a mic onto my jacket, and I try a speed test on the 5G mobile phone I have been lent by EE. I'm getting 260 Mbps – pretty impressive – although the speeds are patchy: even higher if I walk a few yards into the piazza, dropping sharply if I head around the corner.

Now we are connected to Salford, and a voice in my ear tells me they will be coming to me in a couple of minutes for a short hit with presenters Charlie Stayt and Naga Munchetty. There is always a buzz of adrenalin when you do a live TV broadcast. Will I mangle my words, forget a key fact, or even end my whole career by swearing on air? It is a bit like looking over a precipice.

But this is a pretty routine broadcast, and the voice in my ear from Salford tells me the picture and sound are both solid as a rock.

Then, without warning, just a minute before they are due to come to us – the line goes dead.

Nothing. *Nada*. Zilch.

Cue scratching of heads from the engineers and swearing from the correspondent, who asks the traditional helpful question in these circumstances: *What the hell has gone wrong and why can't you fix it?*

None of the usual explanations seem to fit – nobody has pulled a cable out, the Salford control room hasn't cut the feed.

Then there is a dawning realization, which causes acute embarrassment to the EE executives standing and watching.

The SIM card in the Huawei 5G modem has used up its entire data allowance.

It turns out that all the testing done by the engineers over the previous days has chewed through gigabytes of data. Like a profligate traveller watching Netflix on his mobile in the United States, we have breached our plan's limits and been cut off.

Somebody tops up the SIM card, and in a minute we are up and running again. The *Breakfast* producer tells me that fortunately they have found us another slot, and soon I am on air talking to Charlie and Naga and waving my 5G phone around. I explain the significance of the technology we are using, while stressing that it will be some time before many people get their hands on it. All goes to plan: no falling over, no injudicious comments, nothing to worry about.

Except for one thing.

As I come off air and unplug the microphone and earpiece, I am aware of something that has been a feature of several of my recent live broadcasts. As I've been waving the smartphone around, my right hand has been shaking.

The previous October I had been to Jersey in the Channel Islands to report on another connectivity story: the island's achievement in becoming one of the first places in the world to provide a full fibre-broadband connection to every home. In another live broadcast for BBC Breakfast, I stood by the harbour waving a section of fibre-optic cable at the camera.

A few days later, I was forwarded an email sent to the BBC website by a viewer. He described himself as a cellular molecular neuroscientist at the University of York, and said he had watched my broadcast. 'I noticed he had a slight but noticeable tremor in his right hand. This is quite often an early sign of Parkinson's Disease, and I would recommend (if not already) that he seeks advice from his local GP.'

But by the summer of that year I had already been puzzling over a couple of things. I could not seem to stop dragging my right foot as I walked, and my wife had already noticed my right hand shaking a little. I was not particularly concerned but, on the advice of a physiotherapist, booked an appointment with my GP, which took place a couple of weeks before my trip to Jersey and the neuroscientist's letter. The GP had seemed unsure what to make of my symptoms, but referred me to a consultant neurologist at St Mary's Hospital in Paddington.

In the way of these things, that appointment did not take place until four months later, at the beginning of January 2019. It was two days before I was due to fly to Las Vegas for CES (Consumer Electronics Show), the monster annual gadgetfest that is an endurance test for jet-lagged technology correspondents, involving tramping miles through vast hotels in the hope of spotting one innovative product among the AI toothbrushes and self-driving suitcases. After stretching my limbs this way and that, watching me walk back and forth across her consulting room and testing my reflexes with a tap on the knee, the doctor confirmed that I had the symptoms of what she called Parkinsonism. She booked me in for a couple of scans later that month, and in the meantime I set off on my trip to Las Vegas and on to Phoenix, Arizona, to record a radio documentary about the race to build driverless cars.

Although learning that you have what is described to you as an 'incurable degenerative condition' is not a cheerful piece of news,

I cannot say it came as a huge shock, given the warning signs over the previous months, and the work I had done with Dr Google to investigate what was wrong with me. Neither did I see that in the short term it needed to have a radical impact on the way I worked. Yes, the American trip was exhausting – I ate badly and probably had too many late-night beers, but that was par for the course. In the office, my already execrable typing had become worse because of the stiffness in my right hand, but I was coping. There was a slight panic one Friday lunchtime when the BBC's new online production system crashed, taking with it all the scripts I had written for my weekly *Tech Tent* radio programme, and my hand quivered as I set about the slow process of writing the whole lot again in a new document – but then the production system and the scripts came back to life.

In February, as I prepared for another trip to the Mobile World Congress in Barcelona, I realized that the BBC's travel insurance could be affected if I did not disclose that I was suffering from Parkinson's, so I let a couple of my bosses know. A few weeks later, after someone remarked that I was limping, I sent an email to close colleagues telling them about my condition, warning that I'd be less willing to carry the camera tripod – one of the less attractive features of being a news reporter – but still be available for pints in the pub.

But on that May morning in Covent Garden my Parkinson's was still quite a private affair. I had been on medication for a few months, reminded by a smartphone app every few hours to take two tablets which were supposed to alleviate my symptoms. They didn't seem to be having much of an effect, but on the other hand I was not getting noticeably worse. I hurried to the Tube and on to Euston to catch a train to Birmingham to film a new report about the dawn of 5G for the BBC's *Six O'Clock News* and *Ten O'Clock News* programmes. At the station I met Priya Patel, the producer working with me on the story.

Producers play a vital role in the look, feel and content of a news piece, setting up interviews, commissioning graphics, directing filming and discussing with the correspondent the editorial thrust of a report. Priya was one of the best, working mostly with the Economics Editor and proving hugely creative in the tricky task of turning a complex subject into compelling pictures with a clear narrative line. She was also a determined champion of the reporters she worked alongside, lobbying newsroom editors fiercely if there was any sign that they were reluctant to run a story.

But that morning she looked concerned. As we climbed aboard the train she told me she had something she wanted to discuss with me. But our carriage was packed, and we found that our seats were at a four-person table, no place for a private conversation.

Then, at Birmingham International, the carriage emptied out and Priya could finally reveal what was on her mind. She had watched my live broadcast on *Breakfast* from home, then spoken to our news editor, Piers Parry-Crooke, my immediate boss for 20 years and also a steadfast friend. Both had noticed my tremor, which, when I looked at the programme some days later, turned out to have been far more severe than I had realized. Priya had a simple question for me. Had I considered going public about my Parkinson's?

She was pushing at an open door. I had been thinking about just that. But how to do it? Well, in this social smartphone era, the answer was obvious – I had a phone, and my Twitter account had around 170,000 followers. I could do it right then and there.

In the few minutes between Birmingham International and Birmingham New Street I bashed out the following tweet on my phone and pressed Send:

> A couple of people have noticed my hand shaking in my live 5G broadcast today. So seems a good time to reveal that I've recently been diagnosed with Parkinson's. I'm getting good treatment and the symptoms are mild right now – so I'm carrying on as normal. Onwards and upwards!

As we got off the train to go and meet our cameraman, Neil Drake, my phone was already buzzing. Retweets, Likes and sympathetic messages were piling up, from friends, fellow broadcasters, distant contacts and complete strangers. Thirty minutes later, as we arrived at the Birmingham Chamber of Commerce to film our first interview on the potential impact of 5G, my phone rang. It was the BBC Press Office, to say they were already fielding calls from newspapers and could they help?

At lunchtime Priya and Neil were trying to film me walking through the Bull Ring shopping centre talking about 5G – a TV skill that always reminds me of the jibe about Gerald Ford, the US president who apparently could not walk and chew gum at the same time. My walk was repeatedly interrupted by phone calls, one of them from a *Daily Mail* reporter wanting me to give her an exclusive. Somehow, though, we managed to get the piece to camera done and work out a way of illustrating the promised speed of 5G by filming my phone downloading a programme from the BBC iPlayer in next to no time.

As we headed to the BBC's Birmingham studios to edit our package, the responses to my tweet kept coming in. Even Priya got in on the act:

> Having worked with you for a few years now I can confirm today is just the same as always (the usual 5 mins before deadline meltdown expected later).

Now, it is true that, as I have got older, I have found it a little harder to retain my sangfroid as a deadline approaches. The culture of TV news is that you edit right up to the wire, with a perfectionist picture editor sometimes laying the last shot 30 seconds before the director in the gallery shouts, 'Run VT!' I have been known to leave the edit suite once I have recorded my pay-off and wander away, rather than stand behind the editor and producer nervously looking at my watch and urging them to get on with it.

But on this occasion the ever-calm cameraman/editor Neil Drake had everything done by 5.30 and we could head back to London. Sitting on the train sipping gin and tonics from cans, I read through some of the messages I had received. Handily, *Hello* magazine – my first appearance, I think – had collated some of the responses to my Twitter announcement:

Many of Rory's friends were quick to send their best wishes to him after reading his tweet. BBC's Moscow correspondent Steve Rosenberg wrote: 'Sending the very best wishes to a brilliant correspondent. Stay strong, Rory, and good luck with the treatment.' Evan Davis added: 'Rory – you are being showered with good wishes and respect. And deservedly so. Wishing you well as you deal with it.' BBC broadcaster Emma Barnett wrote: 'Onwards indeed', while Channel 4 newsreader Alex Thomson said: 'Wish you well Rory and I am sure we all do at Channel 4. Bravo.'

I have been on Twitter since 2007, and watched it change from a niche network, where geeky folks came to swap ideas, to an essential platform for anybody wanting to know minute by minute what was going on in the world, from celebrity gossip and sports scores to threats of war from the President of the United States.

What I have also seen, as I have voyaged down Twitter's timeline, is the early optimism about what this new form of communication could achieve quickly replaced by gathering gloom.

There was a time when Twitter and its much bigger and more powerful Californian neighbour Facebook were credited with delivering a voice to the powerless, even enabling the Arab Spring, and allowing superstars and their fans or politicians and citizens to talk to one another directly rather than via an old media intermediary. But very quickly the well was poisoned. Trolls and bullies, fraudsters and bigots took to these new platforms with gusto. The Californian tech giants, bent on growth at all costs, seemed unaware or perhaps unconcerned until far too late about the harms they were causing. Today, Facebook is blamed for facilitating everything from the persecution of the Rohingya Muslims in Myanmar to the spread of misinformation and the rigging of elections. Twitter stands accused of giving free rein to white supremacists and Holocaust deniers in the name of free speech. And as for Apple, its critics say its devices have created a generation of zombies, glued to their screens night and day, unable to engage in normal human interaction.

That day, though, was a reminder of the positive side of this social smartphone era that I had been documenting for the past dozen years. Eventually, that tweet announcing my health problems attracted over 1,300 retweets, 40,000 likes and hundreds of messages. With the exception of one fanatic who warned that my Parkinson's was probably brought on by standing next to 5G phone masts, a conspiracy theory we will discuss later, just about every message I received was positive. My phone and my social media feeds had brought me the love and support of an army of well-wishers at a difficult time. It was a day on which the personal and the professional came together. Of course, before the age of smartphones and social media I could have 'come out' about my condition – perhaps giving an interview to a newspaper – but not in the instant and instinctive way I acted that day. What's more, I would not have had the control over my message, or the direct, unfiltered connection with thousands of friends, colleagues and complete strangers – and subsequently a community of people with Parkinson's – that Twitter gave me that day.

A few days later, London's Science Museum got in touch, wanting to get hold of the equipment we'd used in our historic 5G broadcast to add to its collection.

In the following months, as I grappled with other health problems, I began to investigate the role the smartphone, coupled with new artificial intelligence techniques, could play in the treatment of conditions like mine.

Then, in early 2020, as I was starting work on this book, the world changed again. At first, a new virus in China seemed to be just another health scare like swine flu or SARS we in the West could safely ignore. But within a couple of months, that assumption was looking arrogant, and I was locked up at home, like millions of people around the world, in the battle against a global pandemic. It was access to the tools of the smartphone era that allowed me, stuck in my loft office for months, to carry on my job as a broadcaster in a way that would have been impossible a decade or so earlier.

That period took this book in a new direction. The health crisis has magnified both the positive and negative sides of smartphones and social media, bringing people together and offering ways of tracking and perhaps even stopping the virus in its tracks, but also dividing us with an infodemic of misinformation spreading at lightning speed around the globe. It has also enabled me to start reflecting on what I have learned during my years as a technology correspondent, a job where the day-to-day business of chasing stories and competing for airtime leaves little time for long-term thinking.

I grew up in the 1960s and 1970s, a time when technology was exciting but distant and impersonal. It was a period of extraordinary advances, when men walked on the Moon, and Concorde ferried passengers at supersonic speed from London to New York, leaving Heathrow at 9.30 and arriving an hour earlier in time for a second breakfast. But although I watched the Apollo 11 Moon landing on the tiny black-and-white portable TV in our London flat, and marvelled at the futuristic ideas on *Tomorrow's World* (plastic grass? a robot receptionist?), I was confident that I was never going to fly to the Moon or have a robot in my home. The solitary computer at my school filled a room in the Science Block and could only be approached by boys wearing white coats and studying for Physics A-Level – which did not include me. It seemed unlikely that I would ever own one.

Yet by 2020 just about everyone was carrying around a computer with far more muscle than that giant cabinet at school – or indeed those that had guided Apollo 11 down onto the Moon. Technology had become personal, and the combination of smartphones with social media platforms was driving huge changes, both exciting and frightening, in the way we lived. And, as someone with no greater scientific qualification than a barely scraped pass in Physics O-Level, I have been lucky enough to have a ringside seat as this revolution unfolded.

It all started one day in January 2007, when a man in a black polo-neck came on stage in San Francisco to tell us about something he had been cooking up.

Part I

Revolutionary Times

1

'We're Going to Make Some History
Here Today'

It was 11 a.m. on that bright January morning in 2007 as I jogged the short distance from San Francisco's Moscone Centre to my hotel, carrying the precious videotapes of an historic event. That meant it was 7 p.m. in London, and I had three hours to file my report for the *Ten O'Clock News*. Well, not really. As we were using a new and relatively untested way of delivering that report my cameraman and I had set ourselves a deadline of 9 p.m. London time to start feeding our edited package.

My phone rang – I think it was a Nokia N95, very much state-of-the-art back then. It was a producer from the newsdesk in London, for the first time in my memory excited by a technology story. 'We've seen the pictures – it looks amazing! You need to have that phone in your hand for the piece to camera. YOU HAVE TO HAVE THE PHONE!'

I groaned. As ever, London was asking the impossible.

A couple of hours earlier, Steve Jobs had climbed onto a stage and told an excited crowd he was going to unveil three things: a music player, an internet device and a phone – before revealing that they all came in one package, called the iPhone. Cue hysteria.

Now, Apple had a reputation as the world's most controlling company, obsessive about secrecy and delivering the message about new products in its own time and on its own terms. The new phone would not go on sale in the United States until June, and no journalist would get access to it for months. So actually getting my hands on it just hours after it had been unveiled seemed extremely unlikely. But the *Ten O'Clock News* was going to be disappointed if I did not deliver the key shot – the editor might even drop a piece that was always going to be pretty far down the running order. On the other hand, if I rushed back to the conference centre and tried to get my hands on the precious iPhone, I might end up missing my slot altogether, about the most serious crime a TV reporter could commit.

So there I stood on the street, weighing up my options, and casting my mind back to how I came to be in San Francisco at all.

A few months earlier, after I had spent nearly 20 years reporting on business for the BBC, my bosses had suggested a new title, Technology Correspondent, to reflect the fact that many of the stories I was covering involved the impact of the internet on business and society. I was pleased if a little cautious about this appointment: it appeared not to involve any increase in salary, and I had some concerns about the corporation's commitment to the new post. Back in March 2000, the BBC had decided to call me Internet Correspondent, as I was covering so many stories about the dot.com bubble. It was a period when a couple of young entrepreneurs could sketch out an idea – an online store for lightbulbs, a website offering beauty treatments – and find backers eager to give them millions without asking searching questions about their expertise or when they were likely to turn a profit. My wife, an economist, joked that my appointment was a sell signal – and she was right. The bubble burst, dot.com companies melted away and the BBC decided I should go back to being a business correspondent. The internet was over, one of my bosses told me.

A year on, I did manage to get a book out of the experience of documenting the UK's rather brief internet bubble, but as it was published on 9 September 2001 hardly anyone noticed when a rather bigger story came along.

Still, between covering the Marks and Spencer results and the monthly inflation figures, I managed to keep my hand in with a few technology stories. I travelled to South Korea to give *Six O'Clock News* viewers three tales from that hyperconnected nation which seemed to offer a glimpse of the future. We filmed users of Cyworld, a social network which allowed users – and that meant just about every young adult – to create their own idealized world. We visited video-gaming cafés, where young men with bags under their eyes seemed to spend all their waking hours. One had recently died at his terminal. And we covered a citizen journalism project which, we told viewers (somewhat naively), would take power away from the media giants and give it to ordinary people.

And when Steve Jobs came to London to announce the opening of the iTunes Music Store I was there to cover the glitzy event, interviewing both Jobs and Alicia Keys, the star hired to make sure the launch was covered beyond the tech press.

Mind you, I got back to the newsroom that day for the *Six O'Clock News* editor to tell me I had just 1 minute, 45 seconds for my piece, and when I asked how I was expected to fit in the tech titan, the celebrity *and* an outside analyst, her answer was clear. 'Drop the Jobs guy.' That powerful editor has since had a glittering career, and eventually became the executive in charge of Apple TV's European operation.

But by 2007 the Corporation seemed serious about expanding its technology coverage. As a statement of intent the head of the newsroom, Peter Horrocks, decided to send a big team to the Consumer Electronics Show (CES), the vast tech industry jamboree that takes over Las Vegas every January. The idea was that from *Breakfast* to *Newsnight* we would bring our audience the key product launches and dissect the technology trends emerging. This was a big, expensive undertaking. Our 20-strong team occupied a trailer outside the Convention Centre, and a satellite truck drove up from Los Angeles to beam our reports back to London.

But I decided we needed to spend even more money. One company decided long ago it doesn't need to rub shoulders with its peers in Las Vegas – or for that matter at any other grubby trade show. Apple determines when and where to tell its adoring fans about its plans, and that January it was summoning them to San Francisco at the exact same time the world's technology media would be in Las Vegas.

It seemed arrogant. But Apple could afford to be demanding, because at that moment it knew it was the biggest story in tech. Ten years earlier Steve Jobs had returned to the ailing business from which he had been ejected in 1987 and set about breathing new life into it. He quickly spotted that a young British member of the design team, Jonathan Ive, was a kindred spirit, and together they produced a string of products that changed the way we saw computing. The iMac, a design somehow both retro and futuristic at the same time, showed that computers did not have to be boring beige boxes. The iPod became a new generation's Sony Walkman, putting your entire music library into a smart device, with every song available by pressing on its ingenious click wheel. And iTunes, with its store where you could pay to download music, showed that Apple's ambitions stretched beyond computing into the media industries where it had the potential to force radical change.

Even in the bad times, Apple had always had a devoted army of disciples. They saw themselves as superior to the thoughtless masses buying 'Wintel' PCs – the amalgam of Microsoft's Windows operating system and Intel's chips which accounted for about 95 per cent of the personal computing market in the late 1990s. To be a Mac user was to 'think different', as one of the firm's marketing slogans had it: to appreciate good design and a new way of doing things, even if that meant paying quite a bit more. Now, while Apple was still worth only about a quarter as much as Microsoft, its fanbase had broadened, feeding on all the latest rumours in thousands of blogs of what was to emerge next from Apple's Cupertino headquarters. The company's iron discipline about keeping everything surrounding product development secret – even between different internal teams – only served to increase the fevered speculation.

And that January, all the rumours centred on a mobile phone.

Now, at first glance this, unlike personal computers or the music industry, was not an obvious area for disruption. From Nokia to Blackberry, from Samsung to HTC, there were plenty of companies pushing forward with innovative new designs. Finland's Nokia had led the pack in both innovation and market share. Back in 1996 it had launched its first smartphone, the Nokia Communicator, and the phone I was using in 2007, the N95, was the first to make internet connectivity on the move an option for the mass market. Admittedly it was clunky – by the time you had clicked a dozen times through its complex menus to get online you had probably lost patience – but it was a glimpse of the connected future. Others such as Canada's Research in Motion, maker of the Blackberry, were proving that there was a huge appetite in the business community for a device that would let you check your email away from your desktop. So it was by no means certain that Apple, a complete newcomer to the industry, could make any kind of impact.

Nevertheless, I told my bosses, if Steve Jobs was going to unveil a phone, the BBC needed to be there. They agreed to let me take a day away from CES to fly to San Francisco with an experienced cameraman and picture editor, Steve Adrain, for the opening of MacWorld.

We booked into our hotel the night before Apple's show started and immediately did what has since become a key task for any TV crew away from base. Tested the Wi-Fi. For decades, feeding a TV report back to base meant one of two things: travelling to a nearby TV station to use their facilities, or using a satellite truck. Both were expensive but reliable. You would pay a hefty sum to book a 15-minute slot on a satellite just before your deadline, but you could be pretty certain your piece would arrive. Early in my career, a foreign trip involved a lot of people: a three-man crew – yes, almost always men – made up of a cameraman, sound operator and lighting engineer, plus a videotape editor, and often a facilities engineer or two to operate a satellite truck.

You needed transport too: a despatch rider to ferry the tapes around, and sometimes a driver. As a young producer in 1985 I was sent to Paris for a state visit by the new Soviet leader Mikhail Gorbachev. I was working with a very distinguished foreign correspondent who told me to get us a driver, and seemed amused when I asked, 'What – for the whole week?' I ended up handing over to the taxi driver something like £800.

Now, in the digital era, that TV army had been reduced to one person, known as a 'shoot edit'. They would shoot pictures, record audio, then edit the package – and increasingly they were responsible for getting it back to base. By 2007 we were also gradually moving away from expensive satellite feeds to a new essentially free method: feeding the finished package from the shoot/edit's laptop over the internet back to base. In the days of sketchy internet connections this was OK if you had many hours to feed. On one occasion, exasperated by the impossibility of feeding a *Breakfast* report from a Barcelona hotel's congested Wi-Fi, I went round to a friend's house to use his faster broadband connection. It took an hour, but it got there.

What you did not want to do was feed over the internet against a tight deadline. But that is exactly what we were planning to do in San Francisco the next morning: shoot, edit and feed a story for the *Ten O'Clock News* about an event that would not be over until a few hours before the bulletin. Hence the need to test the Wi-Fi. It seemed pretty fast that evening, but who knew how it would perform the following day?

Around 8 the next morning we carried our kit a couple of blocks down to the Moscone Centre, to find a queue outside. We stopped to do a few vox pops, and found people almost bursting with excitement about what they were about to see, for me a new experience at what was essentially a trade show. This was an event where the audience was usually made up of corporate customers, some Apple employees and the media, so apart from the staff you might expect them to be a reasonably sober crowd. But the media now included not just broadcasters and newspapers but dozens of bloggers, many of whom made a living by being endlessly enthusiastic about anything Apple. After all, rumours and general hype about Apple generated clicks, and that meant ad revenue. Many technology journalists at that time may have been a little too starry-eyed about the companies they covered, but the blogging community often had a direct financial interest in their boosterism.

Inside the hall, Steve Jobs appeared on stage in his trademark black polo-neck and jeans, to whoops and hollers. Slimmer and greyer than a few years earlier, with wire-frame glasses, he cut an ascetic, intense figure – a preacher about to deliver the gospel. He waited for the applause to die down, then walked slowly forward for a few paces, his head bowed as if in meditation. He paused, and then began.

'This is a day I've been looking forward to for two and a half years!'

Jobs was a master of the art of unveiling a new product and sounding as if he had discovered nuclear fusion or uncovered a previously unknown Rembrandt. Many have tried to imitate that style, but the difference is that while his products (sometimes) lived up to the hype, theirs never did.

'Every once in a while a revolutionary product comes along that changes everything.' The whooping and hollering grew louder as he expertly teased his worshippers into a frenzy. He took us back to 1984, to the first Mac, then to 2001, to the iPod, to illustrate two such devices. Then he promised to introduce three revolutionary products in the same class.

A widescreen iPod with touch controls.

A revolutionary mobile phone.

A breakthrough internet communicator.

'An *iPod* – a *phone* – an *internet communicator*,' he began chanting.

A tremulous pause.

'Are you getting it yet . . ?'

And then the big reveal, all the more delicious because by now they really were getting it – after all, this was what they'd come for.

These were All. One. Device. And its name was the iPhone.

With trademark arrogance Jobs went on to describe how existing smartphones with their 'plastic little keyboards' were not so smart. Apple, he declared, was going to give the world a leapfrog product that was way easier to use, with no physical keyboard and no stylus. Instead, it would have a revolutionary user interface using the best possible pointing device, the human finger, and an amazing Apple invention called multi-touch. Its software was five years ahead of any other phone – 'It works like magic!'

Suddenly, there it was on screen. The miraculous device . . . It was unlike any phone we had seen: a clean, rectangular slab of glass, with just one button, its purity unsullied by a physical keyboard.

Apple's founder proceeded to put it through its paces. Here's the home button, taking you back to the start . . .

Oooh, went the audience.

Here's the icon for your music . . .

Aaahhhhh!

And now I'm scrolling through your list of albums . . . with just a *swipe of my finger*!

Shattering applause.

Actions that are so commonplace nowadays as to be utterly banal appeared wondrous back then to the crowd in the hall – and I shared in that wonder. The design did indeed appear streets ahead of anything we had seen from another phone-maker, and the graceful ease with which Jobs' fingers danced across the screens making all sorts of wondrous things happen was indeed magical. He even opened Google Maps, found the nearest Starbucks, and made the first call with an iPhone, telling the bemused employee who answered, 'I'd like to order four thousand lattes to go – no, just kidding, wrong number.'

The people looking on and applauding were not just the bloggers and Apple employees who were obviously going to cheer their charismatic leader. In the hall were business partners of Apple, including Bernard Kim, a young executive from Electronic Arts who had just joined the games publisher from Walt Disney. He would go on to work closely with Apple on games for the iPhone from EA and then Zynga, where I met him in 2020 at his San Francisco office half a mile from the Moscone Centre. Looking back at that day, he remembered his excitement at what he saw happening on stage: 'My head literally exploded,' he told me. 'It was actually the cross-section of entertainment, internet and communications all brought together on a gorgeous device with packaging that no one has ever seen before. I really did believe that the iPhone was going to change the world.'

Charles Dunstone was also excited, although rather more British in his reaction. He had visited Steve Jobs and his marketing supremo Phil Schiller the previous summer, intent on sealing an exclusive UK deal for his company Carphone Warehouse to sell the phone that Apple was rumoured to be working on – 'We had heard on the grapevine that they were going to launch it with Vodafone.' He did not get a deal then – that came later – but did get to see a prototype: 'They had a thing that was pretty much like it.' At around £299 it had seemed the iPhone might be a hard sell, Dunstone explained in 2020, looking back to a time when all phones felt effectively free to customers because they were subsidized by the mobile operators. 'But I'd always been a Mac user and an Apple fan. So you couldn't possibly underestimate the potential of what they could do. And they were so confident about it!' And what was unfolding on stage in San Francisco made the Carphone boss feel confident too.

Throughout Steve Jobs' bravura performance my cameraman Steve Adrain was shooting video, and I was trying to get a few stills with my digital SLR camera for a possible blog post. While Steve's footage really captured the mood, my photos were frankly a disaster – I had somehow messed up the settings so Steve Jobs was out of focus.

Years later, I took much better photos of the launch of the Apple Watch, using not an SLR camera but – an iPhone. Photography was just one activity about to be transformed by the smartphone revolution that started that day.

But now we had to get out of the hall, grab a quick vox pop with a British technology pundit and leg it back to the hotel to feed our story to London.

It was a few minutes later that the phone rang with that impossible demand from the *Ten O'Clock News*. My head pounded. I umm-ed and ah-ed. I was going to have to tell the producer that Getting My Hands On An iPhone could not be done.

Then I remembered something. The day before, Apple had offered me an interview after the keynote presentation – not with Steve Jobs but with Phil Schiller. That would be great, I had told the PR person, privately doubting that we would have the time to talk to someone who was unlikely to make it into a two-minute report. I told Steve to continue back to the hotel, spun on my heel and returned to the conference centre. On the way I made a call to make sure that a video journalist working for the BBC technology show *Click* was still there.

I arrived to find Schiller, a short, enthusiastic man lacking the charisma of Jobs, ready to talk – and, yes, *with an iPhone in his hand*. Maybe, I suggested, he could just give me a chance to, ah, *handle* the phone – just a *few* minutes to, you know, get the idea . . . ?

He was fine with that, good old Phil, so I snatched it from him and stood there trying to capture the magnitude of the event in my piece to camera. After a couple of takes, I handed the phone back to Schiller and knocked off a quick interview with him, which of course never saw the light of day. I snatched the video out of the hand of the video journalist and hared back to the hotel. Steve Adrain was just starting to feed our pictures into his laptop to begin editing. He put my new tape in – and I shrieked.

The video journalist had framed it all in a wide shot.

As I delivered my 15-second summary of this Historic Day, clutching the iPhone . . . there was a slightly bemused Phil Schiller standing beside me like a spare part.

Bugger. Unusable – I was certain.

As so often, my skin was saved by a skilled BBC craftsman. Back then we rarely used visual effects in standard news reports, but Steve had one in his locker. He constructed a rectangular box to cover up Phil Schiller, plopped a still of the iPhone in it: job done.

We raced through the rest of the edit, which left us an hour to feed over the hotel Wi-Fi. Steve launched the software that would send the piece to a BBC server in London, and after a few clicks it was on its way. This has become the heart-in-mouth moment where an onscreen clock tells you how long it is going to take for your video to chug its way over the internet to its destination. I have watched in despair as the clock creeps up into the hours, but this time the hotel Wi-Fi was lightning fast, and within 15 minutes the piece was there.

We had done it: delivered a first draft of technology history. Back in Las Vegas the rest of CES seemed pretty lacklustre.

The following Sunday, back in London, I opened the *Observer* to discover its technology columnist John Naughton writing in somewhat sceptical terms about the iPhone launch – and my coverage of it. 'Jobs's launch of the iPhone even made the BBC *Ten O'Clock News*. Business correspondent Rory Cellan-Jones was filmed reverently handling the precious object with the awestruck deference of a medieval peasant confronted with a relic of the True Cross.' I snorted with laughter. Didn't he know how hard this peasant had had to struggle to lay his hands on that holy relic?

But while my report had been well received by my editors, not all viewers had been complimentary. Some had written to the BBC to complain: it was just a plug for a commercial business, or something as trivial as a new phone was simply not news at all. I was invited onto the weekly complaints programme *Newswatch* to defend myself. This was not my first appearance: the year before I had had to defend an interview with the Microsoft founder Bill Gates, even though it had been conducted by the presenter Huw Edwards, not me. The charge was similar: Gates was launching a new Windows operating system – why should we give him the opportunity to promote his business?

Back then, Microsoft was many times more profitable than Apple, and any coverage of its activities resulted in scores of complaints from people who saw it as a powerful and unaccountable monopoly. In 2007, however, the baton was about to be passed. From here on, just about any story about Apple resulted in charges that the reporter was an uncritical 'fanboy'.

So, asked the presenter Ray Snoddy, when *was* a product newsworthy?

I took a deep breath. This was not just any old gadget launch, I insisted: it was a key moment in technology history. Warming to my theme, I went on to suggest that the iPhone was comparable to the Model T Ford – if the BBC had been around back then, surely that would have been a story worth covering?

Afterwards, I thought I had gone over the top. It was far too early to make that judgement about Apple's shiny new device. Across the phone industry executives from Nokia, Microsoft and Blackberry were pooh-poohing the idea that the iPhone had given them something to worry about.

But within a few years, each one of them would be eating their words, as Apple devoured their share of the mobile phone industry's profits.

So, yes, Steve Jobs had been right: 9 January 2007 really was a day when history was made.

2

The Smartphone Revolution

In retrospect it seems inevitable that Apple's iPhone would go on to become the defining product of the early twenty-first century, sparking the smartphone revolution and delivering huge wealth and power to the company which created it. But in early 2007, for all the hype and hullabaloo of San Francisco, many were deeply sceptical about the prospects for Steve Jobs' magical device. Three giant players in the mobile phone industry made it clear that they saw little to worry about, in quotes that would come back to haunt them. Microsoft's bullish chief executive Steve Ballmer, whose Windows Mobile operating system for phones was then enjoying some success, made this bold prediction to *USA Today*:

> There's no chance that the iPhone is going to get any significant market share. No chance. It's a $500 subsidized item. They may make a lot of money. But if you actually take a look at the 1.3 billion phones that get sold, I'd prefer to have our software in 60 per cent or 70 per cent or 80 per cent of them, than I would to have 2 per cent or 3 per cent, which is what Apple might get.

Finland's Nokia had long been the biggest and most innovative force in the industry, and in 2007 it continued to grow, with nearly 40 per cent of the overall market and more than half of the nascent smartphone sector. Even two years later, with the iPhone obviously a hit, Nokia's chief strategist Anssi Vanjoki still thought Apple's phones would remain, much like its computers, a minority interest. 'The development of mobile phones will be similar to PCs,' he told the German paper *Handelsblatt*. 'Even with the Mac, Apple has attracted much attention at first, but they have still remained a niche manufacturer. That will be in mobile phones as well.'

As for Nokia, says Charles Dunstone, the chief executive of Carphone Warehouse, 'We were really really close to them – they were our best supplier. I would be a huge customer for them, so they really were our friends.' Having signed a deal to be the exclusive high street retailer for the iPhone in the UK, Dunstone and a colleague therefore went to see Nokia on one of his regular trips to Helsinki. 'We went there to say, you really have got to watch out, because this iPhone thing is completely different. And they didn't want to hear it.' Somewhat frustrated, his colleague now pitched in. You know why the iPhone's so different? he explained: my four-year-old son can use it. 'And the guy from Nokia said, "We don't want to make phones for four-year-olds."'

But plenty of others were not getting it too. One of the leading technology entrepreneurs in the UK, Hermann Hauser, had worked with both Apple and Nokia for years, and chips designed by the firm he had founded, Arm, were to become standard in the iPhone and indeed all mobile phones. But he too had been unimpressed when he'd watched that presentation in San Francisco: 'Steve gets up on the stage, says I have reinvented the phone, and I thought, Jesus Bloody Christ, what hyperbole! The guy is just beyond belief!' Laughing as he looked back a dozen years later, Hauser recalled how he'd chatted to Nokia executives and they'd agreed that the iPhone was technically far inferior to their devices. 'The number of different frequencies it could do, the battery time, the quality of the voice connection – all that was crap, compared with the Nokia phones. The Nokia phones were much better!'

The Blackberry, the emailing device beloved of Wall Street traders and other high-flyers, was probably the most desirable gadget on the market back then. Its Canadian makers Research in Motion had two co-chief executives, and one of them, Jim Balsillie, had this to say to Reuters about the iPhone: 'It's kind of one more entrant into an already very busy space with lots of choice for consumers. But in terms of a sort of a sea-change for BlackBerry, I would think that's overstating it.'

Mind you, it appears his co-CEO Mike Lazaridis was less sanguine. The authors of *Losing the Signal*, an account of how Blackberry did indeed suffer a sea-change, describe how he watched the Steve Jobs webcast from a treadmill in the gym. 'These guys are really, really good,' Lazaridis told Balsillie. 'This is *different*.' When the iPhone went on sale in June he opened one up and was amazed at what he found inside. 'They've put a Mac in this thing!' he exclaimed. The mobile industry, he realized, was heading in a whole new direction. Phones were becoming computers: ever more sophisticated, tiny computers.

Unlike most senior figures in the mobile phone industry, Mike Lazaridis was a scientist rather than a marketer, and across the Atlantic a young computer engineer was also convinced that he had seen a big moment of change. Eben Upton, later to invent the tiny accessible computer the Raspberry Pi, was working in Cambridge, England on the design of chips to go into Nokia Symbian handsets, Symbian then being the exciting operating system that was going to lay the foundations for the smartphone era. 'We looked at the iPhone webcast,' he remembers, 'and we said, it is going to win. You looked at it and it was just too good. I don't think there were many engineers that didn't know inside six months that it was going to change everything.' Part of it was just about design: 'It was just sexier. It had the Jobs thing: it was designed to be a desirable object, not a functional object. It was very functional, but you could see that it had been designed to be desirable.'

But for Eben Upton and his fellow engineers, the iPhone also signalled a decisive moment in the long-running telecoms industry battle between what they called the bellheads and the netheads: 'the people who saw telephony as being the primary thing in the world, and people who saw packet-switching and computing as being the primary thing in the world.' While old telecoms hands were sceptical that a computer company could hack it in a mobile industry where the operators held the whip hand, the netheads knew this device was one of theirs: 'It was a computer that had a phone in it, rather than being a phone that had some computing functions. The web browser was a real web browser, not some weird thing. It was a *computer*, right?'

Six weeks after the San Francisco launch, I was in Barcelona for Mobile World Congress, the biggest annual shindig for the phone industry, when hotel prices rocket and the Metro workers are usually on strike, making getting a taxi across the city an even more desperate ordeal. There was plenty of talk over the tapas and prosecco of the iPhone and what it might mean for the industry, but no real sense that an earthquake was about to happen. Looking back at what we covered for the BBC that week in 2007, I see that the hot new phones were the LG Prada and the Blackberry 8800, while a Sony Ericsson phone was named best in show. We covered the changing nature of the mobile experience. 'Phones are becoming multimedia entertainment systems,' I wrote, 'with TV on demand, social networking systems and ways of converting every spoken phrase into blogs.' We reported on so-called location-based services, speculating that as I walked down the Ramblas the various bars and restaurants would soon be tracking my phone, and sending me offers as I approached.

But such far-fetched ideas were not yet part of the everyday mobile phone experience. I was still carrying a Nokia, which made surfing the web on the phone more trouble than it was worth. This was the N95, the hottest smartphone of the moment, described by Nokia's Anssi Vanjoki as a multimedia computer. But in truth it was still a phone first – we would have to wait a few more months for the iPhone, the first mobile device to be designed with multimedia computing at its core, to actually go on sale. What's more, the huge cost of using data – especially abroad – meant using services like video calling or music streaming was likely to punch a big hole in your bank balance. As for updating your social network status, Twitter was barely a year old and Facebook was still mainly a campus activity. Most students could not afford a smartphone, let alone a big data allowance.

So let us pause for a moment to consider what our digital life was like in 2007, before the smartphone and social revolution changed everything. It was 16 years since a British scientist at the CERN particle physics lab near Geneva had released into the wild something he called the World Wide Web.

Tim Berners-Lee's creation had succeeded in making the internet, until then the province of scientists and a small band of geeky enthusiasts, a playground for all. Worldwide internet users had topped the 1 billion mark a couple of years earlier, and in the UK 75 per cent of households were online, up from 27 per cent in 2000. That meant all those outlandish dot.com services that went bust when the bubble burst were now becoming viable. Boo.com, the most spectacular victim of the UK's dot.com crash, had burned $150 million on an online fashion website whose home page took nine minutes to download on the average home computer in 2000.

Now in 2007, with more people online and better connections, online retailers like ASOS and Boohoo.com were beginning to thrive, and that year online sales as a percentage of total UK retail broke through 4 per cent.

But there was one big limiting factor on the disruptive power of the internet. Just about everyone was still using it on a computer, either at home or in the office. Even the lucky few that owned a smartphone were rarely using it to shop on the move. Mobile payments services were much talked about, but had not got beyond the pilot stage – except, ironically, in Kenya, where the Mpesa service, which allowed people to send money with a basic phone as easily as sending a text, was about to become a huge hit.

No, mobile phones were still all about texting and making calls. And even though cameras were becoming standard on phones – the first Nokia cameraphone had gone on sale in 2002 – the quality was not great, and they were not much used. If you wanted a decent snap, you needed to have a proper camera with you.

As I was writing these words, I looked at my vast archive of photos stored on my computer. In 2007 I took over a thousand pictures, but in bursts on holidays or at special events, and almost always with a

Canon Digital SLR. Towards the end of the year, I notice, there were a handful of shots with a Nokia N95, including one in November outside London's Apple Store of a happy customer brandishing the first iPhone.

Seven years later, my photo archive shows that in 2014 I took over 4,000 pictures, snapping just about everything every day, from pictures of the dog to portraits of tech tycoons to the launch of the Apple Watch. That year just about every photo was taken with an iPhone 6 Plus, except for a few snapped with the ill-fated Google Glass headset which I was trying out. And by then my 'proper' camera was gathering dust in a drawer. Digital camera sales, which peaked at 120 million in 2010, had by 2018 fallen below 20 million.

In late 2007, you could sense the revolution coming as the iPhone went on sale in the UK, but the wave of change was still not quite ready to crash over the mobile phone industry and the wider world.

There was certainly great enthusiasm in London as queues formed outside the Apple Store, and the first buyers poured through the doors to applause from a chorus line of staff. The Apple fans around the world were more fanatical than ever: when the UK price for the iPhone had been announced a few weeks earlier, a Californian blogger had accused me of 'vacuous pants-wetting' for daring to suggest that it might be a tad expensive compared with rival products. And despite my best attempts to be objective I was very excited about getting my hands on the device I had clutched momentarily in San Francisco. Apple loaned me an iPhone for a week, and afterwards I wrote this in a column for the BBC's staff newspaper: 'Whenever I got it out, it seemed to make me a lot more popular, with crowds gathering to coo and stroke it like a new kitten. Not an experience I'd had with any other phone.'

But the groundbreaking design of the first iPhone concealed some serious technical limitations. There was no 3G, with a slower Edge connection meaning it was hardly worth trying to open web pages when you were not connected to a Wi-Fi network. The camera was very poor with no autofocus or flash and no video capture. And in both the UK and the US Apple had struck exclusive deals with one mobile operator: O$_2$ in the UK, AT&T in the United States. With the iPhone locked to one network, that gave Apple the control over its product it always demanded, but meant the potential audience was limited.

By the end of 2007 over 1.3 million iPhones had been sold, a successful launch but under 1 per cent of global phone sales. Apple was still a minnow, but it was making the rest of the industry sit up and think.

But 2008 would see three developments occur that wrested leadership of what was becoming the world's most important industry from the telecoms firms and handed it to two Californian tech giants.

The first was the arrival on the scene of a new operating system that was eventually to be the bedrock of the huge majority of the world's smartphones. You might have expected the riposte to Apple to come from Nokia, with its Symbian operating system, or from Microsoft's Windows Mobile.

But it was Google, with Android, which became the second Californian upstart to gatecrash the mobile industry's party. Android, an open-source operating system bought by the search engine giant in 2003, was all the talk of the 2008 Mobile World Congress.

Google made it clear that its approach would be very different from Apple's. Not only would it not be making its own phones, but it would also provide Android free of charge to any manufacturer that wanted it, with very light touch controls. Of course, the benefit it hoped to reap was the wider distribution of all of its services, including its hugely lucrative advertising business, on millions of mobile phones. 'We are going to delight users and we'll be able to monetize that,' the Google executive Rich Miner told me at the Barcelona show in a video I filmed on a Nokia N95. We had decided to experiment with blogging and filming with mobiles, although the results did not always impress the audience. 'Give this guy a Steadicam,' wrote one reader. 'It's like the camera's strapped to his head.'

As I summed up Mobile World Congress on my blog, though, I was sceptical that Android would be a huge game-changer: 'There were plenty of new Symbian phones to look at, and Sony Ericsson's first Windows Mobile handset, the Xperia, 1, was rated by many as the best in show. Suddenly talk that existing operating systems would be swept aside by Google's arrival seemed overdone.' And when the first Android handsets appeared later that year, they looked pretty clunky. 'We certainly wouldn't call it sexy,' said the CNET review of the T-Mobile G1. 'Instead, the words "interesting" and "weird" come to mind.'

Nevertheless, more manufacturers kept climbing aboard this new platform and network operators were keen to stock phones with it. Both wanted something to compete with the iPhone – especially those networks that could not stock it – and Android appeared to offer them something flexible and free, unlike Microsoft's Windows Mobile or its later variant Windows Phone.

Meanwhile Apple was not standing still. IPhone users loved the product but wanted more from it – and I was one of them. By March, I was carrying around three phones: a BBC Blackberry which delivered my corporate email, a Nokia N95 to shoot video clips for my blog, and an iPhone which I had bought myself, so determined was I to have one. But this was daft, so I made a video called 'Mr Jobs, Please Improve My iPhone!' and posted it on YouTube. I told Apple's CEO that I needed to consolidate my mobile devices into one and gave him a wish list. I wanted a search facility to find my way through my thousands of contacts, corporate email to replicate what the Blackberry offered, and a camera that had video capture. But most of all I needed 3G. If he could supply all that, I told him, I could chuck away the Nokia and the Blackberry and rely solely on the iPhone.

Now, I do not kid myself that Apple's founder was listening, but a few months later the new iPhone 3G appeared, delivering on most of my needs. A year later the 3GS finally delivered video capture, and then in 2010 the iPhone 4 – widely regarded as the best smartphone ever made – marked the moment when you could leave home with one device that would do just about everything.

But it was another Apple announcement in 2008 that really signalled the start of the smartphone era. Along with the iPhone 3G came a new version of the iOS operating system that included the App Store. The original iPhone had come with the applications chosen by Apple, and nothing else. The ever-controlling Steve Jobs had not wanted users to use third-party apps. But with many users 'jailbreaking' their phones to customize them, Apple bowed to pressure and opened up an App Store where developers could offer whatever they thought would prove popular, albeit under strict supervision – and handing 30 per cent of revenues to the shopkeeper in California. Three months later, Google launched the Play Store for Android – the same idea, but with far more relaxed rules when it came to the kind of apps that could be offered.

A huge new software industry was born, with companies big and small seeing an opportunity to reach millions of customers. In the early days, it seemed that any smart young person could develop an app in their bedroom and swiftly reach an audience. A friend of my son in West London was a perfect example. Sixteen-year-old Edward Bentley made a very simple app called the Impossible Game, and offered it first on Microsoft's Xbox Live Platform. The game, whose graphics were almost laughably basic, involved manoeuvring an orange block past innumerable obstacles and, like another simple game, Flappy Bird, a few years later, it proved extraordinarily addictive. Its creator then reworked it for the iPhone and went through the approval process of getting it accepted for the App Store. Once again, it quickly won a big audience. A little while later, Edward's father answered the phone one evening. He was bemused to hear from an Apple executive in the United States that his game had been chosen as 'App of the Week'. Edward had given his dad's name when registering the app because the rules said you had to be 18 or over.

Eventually, the Impossible Game got to number two in the US App Store chart, and Mr Bentley senior had to open an American bank account to accept the six-figure sum which his son had earned. A decade on, after getting an engineering degree from Cambridge, Edward was working as a software developer – for Apple in Shanghai.

As time went on, though, such stories became rarer, as the app industry got more professional. Soon the default position became that apps were free, sometimes supported by advertising or in-app purchases. For all sorts of businesses, from airlines to banks, from media organizations to retailers, a mobile app became an essential way of communicating with customers or providing them with a service. It was the app economy that made a smartphone the essential tool for modern living, and at the centre of this mobile world were two companies, Apple and Google.

Which left the former mobile phone superpowers high and dry. For a while, developers made apps for Nokia's Symbian, Microsoft's Windows Phone platform and for the Blackberry. But when the audience and the money were all on Android and Apple's iOS it made no sense to keep offering multiple versions of your software.

It was a vicious circle: as fewer apps became available for a Nokia or a Blackberry or a Windows Phone device, their new phones became less attractive, even if the technology in them was sometimes superior to that on an iPhone or an Android. As the giant of the industry, Nokia, began to founder in 2010, the company turned to a Microsoft executive, Stephen Elop, as its first non-Finnish chief executive. I wrote this about the appointment:

> It's a mark of how serious the crisis facing Nokia has become that the company has dumped its chief executive and gone outside Finland for the first time to replace him. The problem is not so much about sales or profits – Nokia is still by far the world's biggest phone manufacturer – as its loss of what you might call thought leadership. The mobile world used to look to Nokia for innovation – now it looks to the likes of Apple, or HTC or Samsung.

The firm was still releasing what looked like innovative new phones running on the Symbian platform, but at the launch of the N8 in London's Excel Centre, the mobile industry analyst Ben Wood summed up the problem: 'The brand is somewhat synonymous with "the phone my dad has".'

Still, with new leadership, the noises coming from the headquarters outside Helsinki, an airy building with a lot of wood and views over a lake that was frozen in winter, were positive. The problems were overstated, the company and its fans said, dismissing the idea that Apple and Google had transformed the industry and insisting it would be madness to drop Symbian or the new MeeGo operating system in favour of Windows Phone or Android.

Then in February 2011, Stephen Elop dropped a bombshell, with one of the frankest and most devastating assessments of a company's prospects any chief executive has ever delivered. In a speech to colleagues which then became public after being transcribed on an internal blog, he compared the company to a man trapped on a North Sea oil rig after an explosion: 'We are standing on a burning platform. And we have more than one explosion – we have multiple points of scorching heat that are fuelling a blazing fire around us.' Then he abandoned the metaphor and came to the heart of the problem: 'The first iPhone shipped in 2007, and we still don't have a product that is close to their experience. Android came on the scene just over two years ago, and this week they took our leadership position in smartphone volumes. Unbelievable.'

It was, I wrote, a hand grenade lobbed into the quiet, understated culture of Finland's mobile giant. And a couple of days later we learnt just how Nokia planned to escape from its burning platform. By leaping onto the Windows Phone rig piloted by Microsoft's Steve Ballmer.

Elop and Ballmer unveiled a partnership which they said would combine Nokia's hardware skills with Microsoft's software. The two sat alongside each other for an interview with me. Stephen Elop explained that the industry had gone through a great shift, 'from a battle of devices to a war of ecosystems – and what we announced today, it's now a three-horse race.' Nokia and Windows Phone would now go to war with Apple's iOS and Google's Android. Elop revealed that he had seriously considered a tie-up with Google, but decided it would be hard to differentiate Nokia phones from other Androids. When I put it to Ballmer that they were way behind in this race and asked how far they could go, typically bullish, he laughed. 'All the way!'

It's now clear that for both men the alliance was one of the great strategic errors. But for a while, it felt like it might work. Nokia brought out the Lumia range based on Windows Phone, and the devices got good reviews, especially for their excellent cameras, which performed far better than those on the iPhone. The sight of one of the firm's new American executives on stage at a Lumia launch trying to channel Steve Jobs by bellowing 'It looks awesome!' may have been unnerving, but sales began to pick up.

By the autumn of 2013, Nokia was celebrating a record 8.8 million Lumia sales in the quarter – though cynics pointed out that 9 million of the latest iPhone model, the 5S, had been sold in just three days. That September, perhaps convinced it was seeing the green shoots of recovery, Microsoft announced it was buying the Nokia phones business for $7 billion. That might have sounded a bargain for a business valued at $150 billion back in 2007, but Nokia investors, who saw their shares rise 40 per cent on news of the deal, breathed a sigh of relief. They had climbed off a platform which, it turned out, was still smouldering. It was a sad day for Europe – in the 1990s Nokia had led the way and helped the continent set the technical standards for mobile phones, but now all the big forces shaping the industry were in the United States or Asia.

For Steve Ballmer, who was about to retire from Microsoft, the deal was the final piece in the jigsaw in his strategy to turn the software company into a devices and services business. But if he hoped it would be a fitting finale to a distinguished career, he was to be sorely disappointed. Just two years later the new CEO Satya Nadella wrote off the entire value of the deal and laid off nearly 8,000 workers, many in Finland. A few years on, the Nokia phone brand was licensed back to a group of the firm's former executives based in offices on the site of the Helsinki headquarters. They proceeded to catch the eye with some delightfully retro handsets which recalled the simple candy bar Nokia phones that had been such hits 15 years earlier. But the aspirations of both Microsoft and Nokia to play a leading role in the smartphone revolution had evaporated.

Meanwhile, the other company which had been so sanguine about the iPhone's arrival was also vanishing into irrelevance. Blackberry sales continued to grow after 2007 – in fact, the Canadian company's revenues peaked in 2011, buoyed by the unexpected popularity of its BBM messaging service, which was a hit with a young demographic, and was even blamed for the spread of the London riots that year. But the business could not seem to decide what it wanted to be. Its core audience, the city slickers who had to be connected to their email at all hours, started turning to the iPhone as Apple wooed big corporate customers. Blackberry remained convinced for too long that a physical keyboard was still essential if it was to hang on to its core audience. BBM may have made it easier to sell new cheaper touchscreen models to younger customers, but they became disillusioned by the poor range of apps compared to what was available from Apple or Android.

In the spring of 2011 I got a real sense of the frustration inside the company about its inability to get its message out, when I went to interview the co-CEO Mike Lazaridis – the man who in 2007 had been more conscious than many of the threat from the iPhone. In a room in a London hotel he was showing off Blackberry's first tablet – Apple had brought out the iPad the previous year, and again its rivals were scrambling to catch up. Lazaridis put the Blackberry Playbook through its paces and all seemed to be proceeding amiably when I turned to something the BBC technology programme *Click* had asked me to raise. Research in Motion, as Blackberry was then called, was under pressure in India and the Middle East, where it had been in battles with governments concerned that its devices were just too secure for their police to monitor.

Perhaps the question I put to him was clumsily phrased. Maybe he thought I was questioning the security of Blackberry rather than suggesting it was too hard to crack – but Mike Lazaridis decided he did not like my tone one little bit. 'Right, it's over, interview's over,' he said testily. 'You can't use that word – it's just unfair. It's not fair. Sorry, we've dealt with this.' He jabbed his finger at the camera. 'Turn that off!' Which we did – but later, along with the Playbook demo, we broadcast the whole exchange.

Blackberry's tablet got a lukewarm reception, and although sales picked up after the price was slashed, it was discontinued a couple of years later. By then Lazaridis and his co-CEO Jim Balsillie had stepped down, and while their successor Thorsten Heins spoke confidently of forging ahead with a new operating system, Blackberry 10, the firm continued its slow decline. Eventually, like Nokia and Microsoft, it got out of mobile phones altogether, though the company made a steady if unspectacular income out of its security software. Which was indeed rather good, just as Mr Lazaridis had implied . . .

Sometimes when I give a talk about the smartphone revolution I put up a slide which illustrates the pace of change that saw an industry completely turned on its head at breathtaking speed.

It is a graphic showing the share of profits among mobile phone vendors from early 2007 to late 2011. At the start, Nokia has around 60 per cent of all the money being made in the industry, Samsung has roughly 10 per cent, and RIM (the Blackberry maker), HTC, Sony Ericsson, LG and HTC are all making decent money.

Apple, of course, is not on the chart at all. But by 2008 its share, coloured blue, is growing rapidly, and by late 2011 it has around 75 per cent of all the industry's profits, and Samsung most of the rest, with a sliver left for HTC. All the rest are now losing money.

Hermann Hauser, who back in 2007 had been so dismissive of the iPhone, says it was Steve Jobs' single-minded obsession which made it work. 'He could put himself into the user's perspective. And because he had this reality distortion field that he managed to create around him, he could imagine what it would be like and what people would really like. This ease-of-use obsession and beautiful design was a killer combination.'

In October 2011, Steve Jobs died, his legacy the single most profitable product ever made and arguably one of the most influential, the iPhone. While sales of Apple's phone surged that year to 72 million, however, that was out of over 470 million global smartphone sales, with Android by far the dominant operating system.

And in all sorts of ways these ever-smarter devices were changing the way we lived and worked. We were using them to play addictive games like Angry Birds, we were reading books and newspapers on them, and just beginning to discover that we could stream rather than own music through services like Spotify. We were checking the weather, booking flights and using satnav apps to find our way to places. And, with the introduction of Siri on the iPhone 4S, we began to talk to our phones.

It was a time both exciting and terrifying. Businesses, governments, hospitals, schools, churches – all were having to come to terms with the changes these magical devices brought with them. But along with the smartphone, and intimately connected with it, another transformative technology was on the rise, promising to shake up the way we communicated and give power to the people. And, once again, it was arriving from California.

3

Facepack: The Rise of Social Media

It is May 2007, and the veteran presenter John Humphrys is introducing an item on BBC Radio 4's *Today* programme, the biggest morning news show in the UK.

> Lily Allen is doing it, the Arctic Monkeys are doing it. Even Prince William is doing it – allegedly – running their social lives on the internet. Social networking – that's how it's described – is the latest big thing on the internet. Sites such as MySpace and Facepack are growing at a lick. And the claim is that it's going to change the face of communication in the way email did a decade ago.

Yes, he did call it 'Facepack', and younger listeners to the *Today* programme – admittedly quite a sparse crowd – may have found the item which followed, a report from our technology correspondent Rory Cellan-Jones, similarly out of touch. The premise was that I, a man in my late forties, was really too old for this social networking malarkey, but was jolly well going to give it a go. I signed up to Facebook, MySpace and something new and outlandish called Twitter – a ridiculous concept where you sent brief text messages to friends telling them you had just had a nice cup of tea.

I then struggled to get friends to join me. There is a passage in the report where I rejoice at finding I have a friend on MySpace called Tom, and my then 16-year-old son breaks it to me that 'Tom' is the founder of the social network and is everyone's friend. And yes, he says, it is a bit sad that I don't understand that.

The piece ends at a networking event where I meet Michael and Xochi Birch, the founders of the very hottest social firm, Bebo, and they agree to be my friends. And such was the influence of the *Today* programme that after the broadcast someone set up a Facebook group called Befriend Rory Cellan-Jones, and I soon had more than 700 'friends', most of whom were total strangers.

In truth, I was not quite as ignorant about social networking as I made myself appear. I had covered the rise of the British network Friends Reunited, which had been sold to ITV in 2005 for £125 million in what had looked at the time an ambitious and far-sighted deal. In 2006 I had done a story on the TV news about schools banning Bebo, which was growing very fast at the time and had produced the first moral panic about social networking. A technology teacher at a private girls' school in Kent told the BBC she was concerned about what pupils were sharing on Bebo – 'some were posting personal details, pictures and even making disparaging comments about the school and its staff.'

But the *Today* programme's interest in social networking was a sign that the phenomenon was breaking out of schools and universities and going mainstream. And yes, while John Humphrys had snorted when his co-presenter Edward Stourton confessed to keeping up with his kids on Facebook, there were growing signs that this might not be just another teenage fad. In the spring of 2007, Bebo and MySpace, each with upwards of 40 million users worldwide, were leading the pack. Facebook, created by Mark Zuckerberg in his Harvard bedroom in 2004 as a campus contact forum, was enjoying a rapid growth spurt now that it had been opened up to anyone, and that spring had over 20 million users. Meanwhile Twitter, created in 2006 by an argumentative bunch of oddballs including Jack Dorsey, had just 50,000 people on board. But the micro-blogging service had one distinctive feature: it was designed for mobile phones from the start, unlike other networks, where everything happened on a computer. In the year the iPhone was unveiled this was a tool fashioned for the smartphone era – though the others would quickly catch on.

After my *Today* programme experiment I quickly became addicted to Facebook, marvelling at how it put me in touch with everyone from long-lost friends to useful contacts for my journalism. The *Observer's* John Naughton – he who had described me holding the iPhone like a piece of the one True Cross – noticed my frenzy of activity:

> Cellan-Jones appears to be spending a lot of time inside Facebook; every time I log in to the site my news feed relates all the things he has been doing. Why? Because I am one of his 'friends' and Facebook thoughtfully keeps me abreast of what my friends have been up to.
>
> Rory has, for instance, been posting videos and photographs, joining groups and leaving intriguing notes about what's happening in his day job and his personal life. I see, for example, that he has joined the 'Mark Kermode Appreciation Society' and 'is home after exhasuting [sic] round of socializing'.

It must have been painful to watch.

But soon I, and it seemed much of the UK technology scene, had decided that Twitter was where the real action was. It was a place where everything was more public, but instead of that annoying bloke from school you hoped you would never see again, you could chew the fat with top tech investors or follow experts on any subject under the sun. And in the early years, when relatively few general journalists were on it, Twitter could make you seem very smart in the eyes of your colleagues and bosses.

One morning in May 2008 I woke early and, as was already my habit, checked my Twitter feed. A number of American bloggers, notably Robert Scoble, were reporting that there had been an earthquake in China. I rang the BBC newsdesk and found that I was breaking the news to whoever picked up the phone. The bloggers had got the news out before the mainstream media or even the US Geological Survey, usually the first source. 'Let's see, as this story unfolds,' I wrote on my blog, 'whether this is the moment when Twitter comes of age as a platform which can bring faster coverage of a major news event than traditional media, while allowing participants and onlookers to share their experiences.'

The social network was also proving its worth as a research tool. When the *Ten O'Clock News* asked for a piece about US researchers claiming a radical advance in battery technology, I puzzled over how to find an expert in this field at short notice. I posted a tweet appealing for help and, 20 minutes later, a press officer at Bath University came back offering a professor who was one of the world's leading authorities on batteries. Soon I was in the car heading to Bath, and the academic proved to be a vital component in my report that night.

Seeing this, colleagues who had been gently mocking my Twitter obsession – 'Why do you want to tell the world you've had a cappuccino?' – started coming to my desk and asking me to tweet when they needed case studies for their stories. As the Twitter audience grew, I tracked down disgruntled airline passengers whose baggage had gone astray or victims of online scams. Eventually they realized that they needed to dive in themselves. 'Can you explain to me how this Twitter thing works?' the BBC's Business Editor Robert Peston asked me one day.

But, intoxicated by the promise of what was still quite a niche activity, I and my fellow technology journalists may have been slow to realize that Facebook was becoming a far more significant and influential force.

In retrospect we can now see that 2008 was the year when Facebook would emerge from the pack to become the most popular social network. But back then it seemed there was all to play for. Yes, in terms of its global audience it did overtake MySpace that summer, but in the United States the music-focused network, which in 2005 had been bought by Rupert Murdoch's News Corp, was still way ahead. That year Bebo was sold to the internet giant AOL for $850 million, making its founders fabulously rich, and surely giving this hugely popular network the financial muscle it needed to compete with Facebook.

So when Mark Zuckerberg came to London in October 2008 it was still far from clear that Facebook was going to end up the winner of the social network stakes. I interviewed him for a *Six O'Clock News* piece – by then even the very conservative editors of TV news bulletins were interested in this geeky 24-year-old – and homed in on his decision to stay independent, unlike MySpace and Bebo. This, remember, was at the very height of the global financial crisis, with shares plunging and banks going out of business by the day. The previous year Yahoo had offered to buy Facebook for $1 billion, and then Microsoft had bought a small stake in the business at what seemed like an extraordinary valuation of $15 billion.

I hit the jet-lagged kid who walked into a cavernous room in London's Excel Centre in sneakers, jeans and a hoodie with what I thought was a series of killer questions. When was he actually going to start worrying about finding a business model and making some money? And what about that Yahoo offer he'd turned down? 'That looks like a mistake now,' I told him sternly. After all, he could have retired at 23.

Up until then his robotic replies had shown disturbing signs of media training, but this time he laughed, and his answer was simple. 'What would I do?' At that stage he was utterly immersed in the building of his business: the idea of giving it up and sitting by the pool all day was, understandably, not enticing. His priority, he insisted, was building an audience, not growing revenue. When I subsequently came to write about the interview I said this sounded to me like a worrying echo of those dot.com days of the late nineties when the accepted wisdom was that you worried about 'eyeballs' on your site, rather than dollars in the bank. I went on to refer to the Bebo sale as a fantastic deal, and warned that 'in the deepening economic gloom, there won't be many more where that came from.' You can't help wondering,' I concluded, 'whether this time next year Facebook's founder will be a little less confident about the wisdom of staying solo.'

It took just a couple of years for me to be proved prescient about Bebo but utterly wrong about Mark Zuckerberg's decision-making. That sale to AOL had indeed been brilliantly timed by Bebo's founders. In the spring of 2010 AOL sold the ailing network, with only around 12 million active users, to a merchant bank for a sum rumoured to be below $10 million. It was eventually bought back by Michael and Xochi Birch for just $1 million. Meanwhile, Facebook zoomed past the 500 million-user milestone in the summer, and when Microsoft's Steve Ballmer came calling with a $24 billion offer for the business, he got a firm no.

In December that year I spent a fortnight in the United States recording interviews for a three-part radio series on the history of social networking. My producer Mike Wendling had done some amazing detective work, tracing the origins of the phenomenon right back to Berkeley in 1973. There, above a record shop, something called Community Memory was born. The world's first computer-based social network involved what one of the founders Lee Felsenstein described as a 'teletype terminal shrouded in a box that I built out of cardboard lined with foam'. People would climb the stairs to type in messages, everything from publicizing gigs to arranging dates – much the same things that we use Facebook for today.

We went on to speak to other influential figures involved in the early social networking scene, from Larry Brilliant and Stewart Brand, who started the Californian online message board the WELL in the 1980s, to the founder of Friendster, Jonathan Abrams, whose 2003 creation had looked set to sweep the world until MySpace and then Facebook came along. But that was programme one: how we got here. By late 2010 we had decided that two businesses had won the battle of the networks, and programmes two and three were largely devoted to Facebook and Twitter.

We arrived at Facebook's Palo Alto headquarters on the day that *Time* magazine announced that it had named Mark Zuckerberg its 2010 Person of the Year. Six years after founding what he called 'thefacebook.com' in his Harvard dorm, he was one of the most famous and wealthy people on earth, and on that day a little too busy to speak to us. We were allowed to wander round the already overcrowded offices in a former factory, spotting posters on the walls. 'What would you do if you weren't afraid?' read one. 'Get excited and make things', said another, an echo of the company's mantra, 'Move fast and break things', which would become notorious a few years later.

If we could not speak to Zuckerberg, one of his most senior lieutenants, Chris Cox, Vice President of Product, was a good substitute, and probably a more articulate and engaging speaker. He gave us this rather brilliant assessment of his single-minded boss: 'He projects this sense that he's in the future and everything's cool there – and he's come a few months back to where you are to tell you everything's going to be fine.' We talked about the bumps there had been in the road, such as the original angry reception for the Newsfeed, the constant stream of updates from friends which had gone on to be the essential feature of the Facebook experience.

'Nobody liked it,' said Cox. 'I remember my entire inbox being full, personal messages to me from friends and family: "Can you please turn this thing off, we all hate it."'

So, I asked, how did you decide you were right and they were wrong?

'If people had stopped using the site,' reflected Cox,

I think we would have reconsidered, but the usage told us people were fascinated. But getting through those first few days, this is a lesson you want to tell anyone who's an artist or a creator or a builder – you just need to have your own vision, and you need to be willing to stick to it in the face of criticism.

Chris Cox insisted the company and its founder were not arrogant, but it seemed to me they had an almost unshakeable belief that they were smarter than the rest of us and could ignore external advice. That worked out fine – for a while.

Our radio programme went on to explore the social network's emerging business model, which saw it offering advertisers the ability to target messages at its users with ever greater precision. My commentary pointed to what would become a matter of huge controversy a few years later: 'Facebook's whole future depends on knowing everything about its members' likes and dislikes and serving them up targeted ads. It's a vision which has already raised serious privacy concerns.' But back then the mood about social networking was largely positive. It was a brilliant new means of communication:

rekindling old friendships, enabling new ones, challenging hierarchies and defying censorship.

That at least was the message when we visited Twitter in its offices in San Francisco, just a few hundred metres from the Moscone Centre where Steve Jobs had unveiled the iPhone nearly four years earlier. One of the co-founders, Biz Stone, told us how the year before he had suddenly started getting lots of messages about a country he had never heard of – Moldova: 'My voicemail on my mobile phone was completely filled up, my inbox was totally overflowing, and they were all asking me the same question which was, "Mr Stone, what was your role in the Moldovan revolts?"'

After a suspect election victory for the Communists in the tiny East European country, a group of young Moldovans got together in a café and decided to start a revolt. They had no access to mass media, just Twitter and Facebook accounts, but after they had used these to spread the word 10,000 people took to the streets in what became known, with a touch of hyperbole, as the Twitter Revolution. The same kind of social media activism was credited with much bigger revolts in Tunisia and Egypt as the Arab Spring got under way. Suddenly, young people armed with nothing more than a mobile phone and a Twitter or Facebook account were shaking up the established order – and politicians were being forced to respond.

'Now, I can tell you that there is no politician in Moldova who doesn't have a Facebook account or a Twitter account,' one of the young Moldovan revolutionaries, Natalia Morari, told our programme. 'They know if they want to know what happens in this new generation – what they are thinking, what they are feeling, what they are going to do – they need to be there where we are presenting most of the time, on social networks.'

This, then, was the golden age of optimism about the impact of these mighty new tools of the digital era. It was as if we had happened on a new land of promise, a place where the old rules and hierarchies did not apply. With a smartphone and a social media account you had as much right to have your say as a prime minister or a chief executive – and if you were a young early-adopter you were undoubtedly more adept than them at using these powerful new means of communication. Just as the Victorians swooned over the arrival of the telegraph, which meant news could arrive as fast as an operator could tap out Morse code rather than at the speed of a horse, or 1950s audiences marvelled at how television gave them a seat at the Queen's coronation, so in the beginning social media on a smartphone seemed magical.

And compared to those earlier communications revolutions, it felt more personal, more creative, more empowering. You might use it just to reconnect with old friends or share pictures of a new baby or a wedding. But you could also stride out onto the global stage social media provided, sharing your emotions, your photos, your theories about the way the world worked, with a huge audience (OK, with your 400 Facebook friends, but they would be sure to pass it on). Instead of ranting to friends in the pub or writing angry letters to the newspapers, you could become a social media personality, or at least engage on equal terms with Stephen Fry or Kylie Jenner or Lionel Messi. Some were already pointing out the dark side of the technology – its addictive qualities, its thirst to gobble up every scrap of data about you so as to sell you things. But in the early days there was still very little advertising on social media, and the companies seemed like scrappy Davids rather than bullying Goliaths.

And the impact of these tools went far beyond just politics and revolutions. Back home in the UK I kept coming across people whose lives appeared to have been transformed by the technology. Let us meet two such people: a woman who helped save the home of one of Britain's greatest wartime achievements, and a Lake District shepherd who became a best-selling author.

It was in the summer of 2008 that I first met Dr Sue Black. She had already been on quite a journey. At 25, she had been a single mother with three children and no job, living in a women's refuge, and now she was head of the computing department at the University of Westminster.

We met at Bletchley Park, the wartime codecracking centre near Milton Keynes in Buckinghamshire then in a state of sad disrepair. This was the place where the computing pioneer Alan Turing had first put some of his ideas into practice in the gargantuan effort to decode German messages. For many years Bletchley's vital role had been kept secret, but it was emerging from the shadows and its place in the history of the war and of modern computing was being recognized.

Sue had first visited it five years earlier and been amazed to hear about its history, and in particular that 80 per cent of the 10,000 people who worked there had been women. So enthused had Sue been that she started an oral history project, persuading some of the women codebreakers to tell their stories for the first time.

Then in 2008, at a reception at the site, two things happened. The director of the charitable trust that ran the museum told Sue its finances were in such a bad way that it might have to close. Then she walked around with one of the veterans who had worked there, and he told her it had been estimated that Bletchley Park's work had shortened the war by two years, saving millions of lives.

'I just stood there thinking: this place might close,' Sue told me: 'I've got to do something about it.' She'd mulled over getting together a petition, or maybe a letter to *The Times* from fellow computer scientists at universities. Then she'd decided to ring a couple of media contacts, including me.

I knew a bit about Bletchley Park and liked the sound of the story but, according to Sue Black's account, I'd told her I was not convinced I could sell it to editors. Then, she says, I rang back a few days later and said that if that letter could end up in *The Times* it would provide the story with a suitable hook. And with a phone call from me to persuade the paper to publish, this most old-media of approaches ended up being the launchpad for the campaign. I filmed the dilapidated huts where the codebreakers had worked, interviewed Sue and dug out some archive footage. The story, carried on BBC radio, TV and the website, made quite a splash, but the news caravan moved on, and the campaign might have just faded away.

But a few months later, Sue Black woke up to the power of social media. There was a Save Bletchley Park Facebook page, and the campaign began using Flickr to share images. But it was Twitter that was to become the key weapon.

Like me, @Dr_Black, as she was known on Twitter, had joined what we then called the micro-blogging service in the summer of 2007, while not really seeing the point of it. Then one day, at a conference in London, she was sitting in the front row when the speaker, a young blogger and budding social media consultant called James Whatley – or @whatleydude – asked people to put their hands up if they used Twitter. Sue raised her hand, as did her neighbour Jonathan Raper, who went by the handle @madprof. 'I turned to him and said, "Yes, but it's a bit shit, isn't it?" He said, "No, no – it's amazing!" Sue had not installed it on her mobile phone, so the mad prof explained that she needed to download an app called Tweetie which would transform her experience. He showed her all the conversations he was having with people across the tech community. 'It was a lightbulb moment for me. I thought, I can use this for the Bletchley Park campaign . . .'

She hooked up with two Twitter early adopters, Mike Sizemore – @sizemore – and photographer and blogger Christian Payne, known as @documentally, and took them on a tour of Bletchley Park. 'I really wanted people that were interested in it to see what it's like there and get really excited about it, because I knew then that they would go out and just talk about it to everybody, and they had much more of a following than I did.' It worked: they set up the @bletchleypark account and showed Sue how useful hashtags could be to gather people around a topic. By then, Twitter was where much of the computing world was hanging out, along with influential geeks such as the actor and writer Stephen Fry.

One day in February 2009 Sue noticed this tweet from Fry: 'OK. This is now mad. I am stuck in a lift on the 26th floor of Centre Point. Hell's teeth. We could be here for hours. Arse, poo and widdle.'

The actor's elevator incarceration was an early Twitter moment, and inspired Sue Black to send him a direct message about her campaign.

I just thought Stephen Fry must be interested – I know he loves technology and history. So I checked his profile and luckily he was following me. I sent him, I think, three direct messages that night just basically saying, if you get involved you could make a massive difference, please help.

The next day the actor tweeted a link to her Bletchley blog and the impact was startling. 'On my blog I was getting about fifteen hits a day, and one tweet from Stephen Fry and I got eight thousand hits that day. And that day I was the most retweeted person in the world!' Back then Twitter was quite a small world with around 20 million users, but in some ways that made it a more effective, focused and less hierarchical community. These days celebrities such as Stephen Fry might be less likely to follow or engage with an obscure academic.

From then on the campaign gathered pace. Fry visited Bletchley Park, and I went along, as did Christian @documentally Payne, who tweeted, filmed and blogged every moment. The moment the actor turned up for what was supposed to be a private visit he was spotted by a member of the public who tweeted about his presence, and the whole day turned into a major social media event.

A few months on, a tweet from Sue Black about some historic papers by the computing pioneer Alan Turing which were up for auction and in danger of being lost to Bletchley Park was spotted by a Google executive in California. He helped raise some of the cash to buy the papers, and the search engine giant then lent its considerable weight to the wider effort to renovate the Bletchley site. Before the campaign had got under way Bletchley had been turned down when it sought help from the National Lottery Heritage Fund. But in October 2011 the Fund awarded the site a grant of £4.6 million, and its press release announcing the news came with a quote from Stephen Fry calling it 'a monumental triumph for the Bletchley Park Trust'. 'Not only did these people change the very course of history by helping to secure the Allied victory, thereby quietly and modestly providing us with the free world', said Fry of the wartime codebreakers, 'they also gave birth to the Information Age which underpins the way we all live today.'

The threat to this extraordinary piece of wartime and computing history had been lifted. 'I think if we hadn't had Twitter it wouldn't have worked,' says Sue Black. 'We just couldn't have done the things that we did.'

If social media could supercharge a campaign, the new technology could also give a voice to individuals far from the centre of things.

James Rebanks was most certainly not a celebrity or an influential geek when smartphones and social media came along. He was a shepherd, tending a flock of hardy Herdwick sheep on the small farm he had inherited from his father in the fells of the Lake District, east of Keswick.

It was a tough and only marginally profitable existence, although he did have another income from consultancy work for UNESCO. A rebel who hated school and left at 16 with two GCSEs, he later discovered a love of literature and ended up studying history at Oxford in his mid-twenties. But he returned to run the farm, and to this day he is still far from enamoured with the modern world and its technology. When the iPhone came out in 2007 he remembers thinking Apple was 'a weird cult' and the worship of its products insane and nonsensical. 'I'm not very interested in new technologies, which I have always thought more often than not make things worse,' he says. 'We rarely think through the effects of technologies, and have a childlike faith in "disruption" being a good thing.' He points to the adoption of technologies by farmers in the twentieth century, claiming that while they have fed billions of people they have also trashed the planet. As for social media, he had thought 'it sounded like people filling the airwaves with facile gibberish – it seemed to be about the Kardashians or whatever and nothing to do with me.'

That changed in 2012 when some friends suggested he use Twitter, and he acquired the handle @herdyshepherd1. For someone so contemptuous of the very idea of social media he appears to have plunged in with gusto.

His early tweets, most of them featuring excellent photos of sheep and the landscape, make it clear he was a man on a didactic mission to tell his followers about farming and its role in preserving the countryside. 'This time of year is all about maintaining the condition of our ewes, whilst they are in lamb,' was his first message that January. He must have had a response. A few days later he tweeted this: 'It's really encouraging that people are interested in what we do. At times it can feel that many people would rather we disappeared.'

What he had to share was both beautiful and compelling: a daily picture of his working life through the seasons – the hard times when the snow came and dozens of his ewes were in danger, the sheer exhaustion of lambing through the nights in April, the exhilaration of leading his flock up onto the fell for summer grazing. In between came an often passionate and angry view of hill farming's place in modern Britain, with occasional clashes with those who saw it either as antiquated or, in the case of the *Guardian* columnist George Monbiot, as an active threat to the environment of the Lake District, reducing it to a treeless waste. At first, with no phone signal on the fells, he tweeted from home in breaks in his working day. Then, as reception improved, he was snapping photos on his iPhone of everything he saw as he roamed the hills.

Rebanks soon had thousands of followers, including me. In 2013 the American magazine the *Atlantic* spotted him and asked him to write something about being a tweeting shepherd. 'Wow @ herdyshepherd1 has made it across the Atlantic!', I tweeted, and he replied, 'It's the internet Rory, it's brilliant, u can send emails and everything!' His article, bylined with his Twitter handle because he still wanted to remain anonymous, described how despite his distrust of technology he had come to realize what a powerful combination a smartphone and a social media account could be:

> I was a little behind the curve on getting an iPhone, and accepted it reluctantly as a free 'upgrade' when my perfectly fine old mobile died after years of good service. I hated the cult of Apple: I was going to resist.
>
> But whatever I wanted to happen, I suddenly had a camera and Twitter app in my pocket whilst I worked. And though it took me a while to realize it, I had the tools to connect to thousands of people around the world.

The article brought a new surge of followers, while also revealing that here was a gifted writer with something to say about a world which was both fascinating and little understood. Publishers took note.

In 2015 I travelled to his farm in the Lakes for an exhilarating day, spent mostly in the trailer of his quad bike, filming him for a *BBC Breakfast* piece. 'I didn't really understand how Twitter worked at first,' he told me,

> but quite quickly I realized that there is a huge number of people that are really interested in what we do. It is an interesting story and that's been shown through Twitter. I think people really do want to know about where their food comes from and about farming.

If anything, his sheepdogs were becoming even bigger stars. By now he was experimenting with Twitter's video platform Vine, and when he showed his collie Floss with her new puppies, 600,000 people tuned in.

By then, Rebanks was a published author. After that *Atlantic* article came out Penguin had won a bidding war for his memoir *The Shepherd's Life*, and the book was winning critical acclaim and featured as Radio 4's Book of the Week. It went on to sell more than half a million copies and was translated into 16 languages, setting the tweeting shepherd off on a new path. He stayed on his farm, but he was becoming a public figure with a burgeoning literary career and a role in lobbying on countryside issues. It seemed that the smartphone social era, which at first he had viewed with some contempt, had proved a liberating force.

Five years later, I visited him again. Over the previous years he had fallen in and out of love with social media, leaving Twitter and then returning on several occasions. Earlier in 2020, when I had contacted him about this book, he had seemed ready to abandon it altogether. 'I think on balance that social media has been a disaster for the human race. A disaster in politics. A disaster in environmentalism,' he wrote to me.

What on earth were we thinking? That it would be great if we all had a voice and could publicly argue every hour of every day? I think we had optimism bias – that we would be listening to wise and expert voices – whereas it is really our racist uncle, our selfish cousin, and our misogynist neighbour given a megaphone. I am struggling to stay on it, and try to filter out the nonsense and focus on the good people and the good stuff that it can do.

But on my visit in August, as his new book *English Pastoral* was published, he was in a far sunnier mood. This love letter to his Lakeland farm, and sometimes angry manifesto for a return to a greener form of agriculture, put him in the public eye again in the year when the pandemic had made food security a pressing issue. By now, Instagram seemed to be his preferred platform, a place where he could post glorious pictures of the farm, illustrating the way he was transforming it with different livestock and more careful management of the land, without getting into arguments. Those still flared up from time to time on Twitter, but his main focus on social media now was talking about and promoting his new book and its message about the future of food production in Britain. His wife Helen had also become something of an Instagram celebrity with her account @theshepherdswife, again posting idyllic photos of the farm and the family with occasional ventures into the campaign to protect British agriculture. 'Helen's the future,' Rebanks told me with a grin.

Together they seemed to have worked out a smarter way of using social media: aware of its dark side, but also conscious of its power as a platform where voices from a small hill farm on a Lakeland fell can be heard around the world.

For much of the first decade of the smartphone social era, a sense of optimism about what this technology could do for us prevailed. Yes, there were plenty of lurid headlines about our growing obsession with our phones, and the amount of time young people in particular were staring at their screens or interacting on social media rather than in real life. But then again, the same concerns had been expressed about the arrival of the telegraph, radio and television. What this ultra-connected world, where economic power depended on the collection of vast amounts of data, implied for the privacy of individuals was a different concern. But then again that appeared to be a niche interest. 'Privacy stuff does not resonate with "normal" people,' the Californian tech blogger Robert Scoble told the BBC in 2010 after one of many Facebook privacy scandals.

What did become rapidly clear was that all of the wealth and all of the power in this new era seemed to be concentrated in the United States – or rather California. That was where the Facebook empire was based, and where Instagram and WhatsApp got started before they were gobbled up by Mark Zuckerberg's firm and housed in his sprawling Menlo Park campus. A few miles down the freeway was the Mountain View headquarters of Google. At first it had stumbled in the social media stakes, with Google+ and Orkut ground under the wheels of the Facebook juggernaut. But everyone seemed to forget it owned YouTube, a hugely influential platform where billions came to consume and create, and as the owner of Android it was one of the two key players in the smartphone industry. The other was of course Apple, across in Cupertino. It never mastered social media, but the iPhone was transforming industries from music to transport to newspapers and turning its creator into a trillion-dollar business.

Britain, by contrast, was wondering how it could thrive in this world beyond offering a European launchpad for the Californian giants, who would offer some jobs but pay very little tax. The country that had been a pioneer in computing after the Second World War and again briefly in the 1980s had struggled ever since to build a technology company or product to take on the world. But in 2011 an unlikely world-beater was about to take off, borne aloft on the wings of social media.

4

Raspberry Pi: Can Britain Build a Computer?

In May 2011, two visitors from Cambridge came to see me at my office at the BBC's Television Centre in West London, in the mistaken belief that I had some influence over the workings of the Corporation. In the 1980s the BBC had partnered with Acorn Computers to create the hugely successful BBC Micro, which introduced a whole generation to computing. Now, David Braben and Eben Upton thought the public service broadcaster might be willing to get behind a little computer with similar if more modest ambitions. They called it Raspberry Pi, and a group of Cambridge computer scientists, academics and entrepreneurs had been trying to get it off the ground for half a dozen years.

What happened in my office that morning in 2011 was an illustration of how powerful a combination of smartphones and social media could be. But before we find out more about my two visitors and their plan for a new British computing device, let's remind ourselves how unlikely it seemed back then that they might succeed. After all, it was quite some time since the UK had been at the forefront of innovations in computing.

As we have seen, the major companies that shaped the smartphone social era were either American or Asian. In the earlier stages of the mobile communications revolution, Europe had been a major force, perhaps even the leader. Manufacturers like Finland's Nokia and Sweden's Ericsson set the pace in making innovative phones, and the UK's Vodafone and France's Orange were among the most innovative mobile phone operators when it came to introducing new services. The United States was a laggard in areas like SMS – one reason Twitter took off when it did was that Americans were finally getting used to texting – and in mobile payments.

But after 2007 Apple, South Korea's Samsung and then a clutch of Chinese companies quickly outpaced the Scandinavian manufacturers. By 2012, Samsung was in the lead ahead of Apple, and together the two had around half the total market. China's Huawei and ZTE and Japan's Sony made up the rest of the top five. With Apple and Google now dominating the software and services on mobile phones, mobile operators like Vodafone had a lot less power and far skinnier profit margins. As for social networking, that came with a uniquely American flavour, unless you were Chinese, with services such as WeChat soon proving hugely popular and innovative in a country where Facebook and Twitter could not operate. For technology journalists this shift in power was clear in the constant refrain from PR people in Europe – 'Can I get back to you after California wakes up?' Most stories seemed to involve companies based on the West Coast – or later Shenzhen in China – and while they employed plenty of people in London, Paris or Berlin it was clear where the influence lay.

For Europe, and the UK in particular, this was a time of economic anxiety and a growing technology inferiority complex, summed up in the often heard question: 'Why can't *we* build a Google or a Facebook?' The UK, while short of major technology businesses of the stature of Germany's SAP or Siemens, did have one contender to be a world-beating company in the smartphone era. Cambridge-based Arm, spun out of Acorn Computers, was a chip designer whose technology rapidly became standard in most mobile phones. But later it, like many other promising British technology firms, was to lose its independence.

The UK also had Europe's most vibrant start-up scene, increasingly clustered around London's Old Street roundabout, rechristened Silicon Roundabout. But while the volume of venture capital invested in the UK was many times that available to French or German entrepreneurs, there were few signs that it was generating businesses that could compete globally with the likes of Google or Facebook. One reason was that the amount of capital available to get smart ideas off the ground in Silicon Valley was of another magnitude altogether, compared to anywhere else on earth.

The story of Hailo exemplifies the problem. In 2013 I wrote about this business, started in London two years earlier by a group of entrepreneurs, including three cab drivers, to build a smartphone app which 'allows you to virtually hail a cab'. They had just raised another $30 million and unveiled plans to launch in New York and Tokyo. The chairman, an American, Ron Zeghibe, told me he had seen the venture capital scene in London transformed over the previous 20 years, with plenty of money now chasing good ideas. 'So cabbies and capitalists coming together to build a global business from nothing inside two years,' I wrote. 'Maybe London's ambitions to be a rival to Silicon Valley aren't so bonkers after all.'

In all, Hailo raised something like $150 million from venture capital backers, a huge sum for a UK start-up. But it never did become a world beater, because something called Uber came along and swept it away. The California-based 'ride-sharing' app – I always found the idea of the 'sharing economy' somewhat ludicrous – ended up raising over $25 billion, enough for it to go on losing money for many years while it raced around the world conquering new cities, whether their municipal regulators liked it or not. Now, Hailo made plenty of mistakes, but competing against a rival with such deep pockets was always going to be a virtually impossible task.

But there was one UK tech start-up that did end up making a global impact in this era. It did not have access to vast amounts of capital – indeed, it never went near the offices of any venture capitalists, relying on a few thousand pounds from its founders to get off the ground. It was not even designed to be a business – more an educational project which took an unexpected turn.

This was the Raspberry Pi that Eben Upton and David Braben came to tell me about in 2011. Its story might at first seem a diversion from the main narrative of this book about the rise of the smartphone and social media. But it embodies some of the optimism of the era, a feeling that technology was for everybody and could be a life-enhancing force. And without the combination of a smartphone and the social media platform YouTube it might never have taken off.

Until the twenty-first century, personal technology was not for children, or at least not grown-up communication devices such as mobile phones or laptop computers. I came back from a trip to Finland in 2000, having filmed a report with a family where everyone – mum, dad and two children – had their own Nokia phones. This was considered so outlandish by the editor to whom I pitched the story that at first she was unwilling to run it.

At the beginning of the century, just a third of UK adults owned a mobile phone, and only a quarter of homes were connected to the internet. But in 2011, the UK's communications regulator Ofcom put out a report entitled 'A Nation Addicted to Smartphones'. It said that nearly half of all teenagers owned a smartphone, a higher proportion than adults, and what it called 'generation app' was using these powerful devices to play games, take pictures, update their social networks and myriad other things.

This may have appeared to be a new computer-literate generation – three-quarters of homes now had an internet connection – but there was a growing concern in the technology industry that this was not the case. There may have been a few bedroom app developers, but the vast majority of teenagers had no idea what was going on behind the screens of their smartphones and little interest in finding out. In fact, the video games entrepreneur Ian Livingstone had co-authored a report called 'Next Gen', warning that there was a severe shortage of the kind of computing skills the UK needed. He put a lot of the blame on the education system. 'Children had become users of technology but had no idea how to create their own.'

But on that May morning in 2011 David Braben and Eben Upton outlined their plan to change the way children saw computing. Each of them had seen at first hand how big a gap there was between the UK's aspirations to be a leading player in technology and the reality of a generation emerging from schools without the skills to make that happen.

Braben was a pioneering figure in the UK's games industry. As a Cambridge student in the early 1980s he and a fellow undergraduate had built Elite, the world's first 3D space exploration game. He had stayed in Cambridge and started a games business called Frontier, which had been successful enough to allow him to invest in other companies as well as continuing to run his own business. Upton was younger but had followed a similar trajectory, reading computer science at Cambridge and making a decent slice of money – 'enough to buy a house' – during his postgraduate research by designing games for mobile phones. He had gone on to work at the Cambridge offices of the US chip developer Broadcom, and to get an MBA from the city's Judge Business School, but it was a short period as an academic that was to open his eyes to a problem in computing education. As Director of Studies for Computer Science at St John's College, Cambridge, it was his job to select candidates aspiring to study at one of the world's most prestigious universities, and one of the cradles of modern computing.

But here was the problem. While you might have expected an army of eager and talented young people to be clamouring for places, that just was not the case. 'In 2004, I went into the tutorial office to get my stack of application forms, and it was that thick,' he explained many years later, almost pinching his thumb and forefinger together. 'You'd expect a brick. And in 2004 I admitted everybody who was any good – and that was scary.' The whole point of an elite course at an elite university was to select not just good candidates but exceptional ones. 'And 2004 wasn't even the bottom of the curve. It got worse and worse.'

Meanwhile, further down the talent pipeline, David Braben was trying to recruit exceptional software developers for his games business and experiencing the same problem. 'We noticed that the number of graduate applicants to select had really dropped, and not just from Cambridge.' And this was not just about one games company's recruitment issues. As the UK entered the smartphone era and the app economy took shape, it was becoming clear that the country was severely lacking in the skills that would be needed.

Braben thought he knew what was to blame: the rise of a subject called ICT in the secondary school curriculum. ICT was meant to give teenagers a broad range of computing skills, but it was not a specialist subject, and they were unlikely to emerge from it with any knowledge of coding. Critics said ICT was about little more than learning to knock up a PowerPoint presentation or use other components of Microsoft Office, and there was a growing chorus of complaint from both the technology industry and specialist teachers calling for change in the classroom.

David Braben remembers that at the time his nephews were of an age when they wanted to learn about computers. 'And I thought it was really depressing that the best solution was to get a BBC Micro down from my loft and set it up.'

That exceptional computer was another thing he and Eben Upton had in common. For Braben it was the platform on which in 1983 he and his fellow Cambridge student Ian Bell had built Elite, launching his career in games. For Upton, it was the computer he had bought in 1989 aged 11 with savings from birthdays and Christmas presents. 'It was second-hand, very beaten-up – you had to beat it to make it work! – but I loved that machine.' And for him too the Micro opened up a path to a career in computing.

At the founding meeting of Computing at School, a group set up to press the case for change, Braben found himself talking to another Cambridge luminary, Jack Lang, a computer science professor and entrepreneur, who had been involved 20 years earlier in the development of the BBC Micro. They agreed on the need for a project to get schoolkids interested in coding, and soon a nucleus of Cambridge people, including Eben Upton, had assembled around the idea.

At first, the plan was to create some kind of software for schools, and when Jack Lang suggested a piece of hardware, a successor to the BBC Micro, Braben admits he was a bit sniffy. 'I thought, that's an interesting idea, but quite challenging.' After all, developing computers is a not-inexpensive business. But Eben Upton, by then working at Broadcom with its plentiful resources, took up the challenge. He remembers an email chain with the title 'Redo the BBC Micro', and says the idea had been kicking around the university's computer lab for some time.

The email group began discussing a name. In a technology world where Apple, Blackberry and Orange were familiar names, Raspberry seemed a possible – and while the BBC Micro had used the Basic programming language, Upton's prototype device was built on its modern equivalent, Python. So, Raspberry Pi.

For a couple of years, while Upton was immersed in his MBA, nothing much happened – except that the Broadcom chip which was to be at the heart of the Pi became more sophisticated, using technology from Arm, which of course had been born out of Acorn, maker of the BBC Micro. But by May 2011, things were beginning to move again. By then the prototype device was about the size and shape of a USB stick; it looked like a scrap of circuit board but had ports to plug in a TV or monitor, a mouse and a keyboard and, unlike the BBC Micro, which had been an expensive product, the team wanted it to retail for $25 or around £15.

The hope was that the BBC might lend its name and its support to the project, but they were finding, as have so many, that dealing with the public service broadcaster these days was something of a bureaucratic nightmare. Along with Pete Lomas, another key figure in the project, Eben had a series of meetings with the BBC Research and Development team in Manchester. 'They were very excited, but unable to consider putting their name on this thing.' David Braben was also losing patience: 'I found the BBC to have so many committees needing to sign off on things, it felt like I was wading through treacle.'

I had visited Braben at Frontier in Cambridge that April to film a report on one of his games, which had been nominated for a BAFTA. Afterwards we got talking about the state of computing education, and he told me about the Raspberry Pi. It was a few weeks later that he and Eben Upton pitched up at my office, hoping that I could help them find a path through the BBC treacle. I told them that even if

I had any influence – and I did not – the BBC was a much more cautious beast when it came to commercial projects than it had been back in the 1980s. Even the BBC Micro had been quite a controversial experience for the corporation, with the somewhat combustible computing tycoon Clive Sinclair angry that Acorn had been chosen as a partner rather than his much-better-known Sinclair Research. More recently, an online educational venture called BBC Jam had been shut down after complaints from commercial businesses that it was distorting the market.

So the BBC Nano, as they wanted to call it, was never going to happen. What I could do, however, was report on the project. At that stage this was not a story that would make it onto the TV news bulletins, so I could not call up a camera crew. Instead, I got out my iPhone and filmed David Braben giving a quick demo of the Raspberry Pi. The video was very simple, an unedited single shot with me off-camera panning between him and the device. 'It's a little tiny device that is a computer on a USB stick,' Braben explains.

> It's got HDMI on one end, USB on the other end, and the idea is you plug it into an HDMI TV, you can plug in a USB keyboard and use it as a computer to be able to learn programming – to be able to run Twitter, Facebook, whatever – but also to be able to understand the whole process of programming.

He goes on to answer a couple of my questions, explaining the wider mission and his concerns about computing education. When I ask how soon the Raspberry Pi will be in every child's hands, he says that will take a while, but 'we hope that something will be rolled out within twelve months.'

I said goodbye to both of them, uploaded the video to my YouTube channel, and embedded it in a BBC blogpost about the Raspberry Pi project. Later that Thursday, I clicked on my YouTube page and was surprised to find the Raspberry Pi video had already had over 10,000 views.

I had started using the video-sharing service in 2006, just a year after it was founded, and uploaded a mixture of family and work stuff, from cheesy ski holiday videos to mobile phone launches. Most got seen a couple of hundred times, although my biggest hit at that point had been a review in 2007 by my nine-year-old son of a laptop aimed at children in the developing world, which had nearly 19,000 views. But the Pi video was going viral with a vengeance. Twenty-four hours later it had topped 130,000. My blogpost was getting comments, too, some applauding the ambition of the project, others sceptical, but after the Slashdot tech site linked to the video most of the traffic was going to YouTube rather than the BBC.

The viewer count continued to climb. By the end of the weekend more than 400,000 people had seen the video, and quite a few of them were getting in touch with the Raspberry Pi Foundation, wanting to know more, wanting to get involved. 'I was getting one email a minute at least, if not an email every ten seconds,' says Eben Upton. 'I mean, it was a *massive* spike of emails.'

A couple of years later he was to describe this as the 'Oh, shit' moment: 'We had to figure out how to make what we promised to do actually true.' For David Braben, it made everything much clearer. 'That discussion with you and the video was quite instrumental in us just saying, right: we'll just go for it. And we'll use our own name: Raspberry Pi, not the BBC Nano.'

Going for it meant a project which had lived up until then on goodwill and unpaid work now needed to raise some money. They scrambled together just over £100,000, with Jack Lang, David Braben and Eben Upton contributing the lion's share out of their own pockets, and a few wealthy individuals in Cambridge chipping in too. The other key contribution was that Eben's wife Liz, a freelance editor and food blogger, came on board and started a blog and a social media effort. Swiftly, a community grew up around the Raspberry Pi which was to prove crucial to its success. 'Once you had published that blog post about the prototype everything went nuts,' Liz Upton told me, referring to my BBC article. Later, as the charity did not want to spend money on customer support, its online forums became the place to go for any technical help. But at first their website and the Twitter account were a focus for those who wanted to shape the project.

'People were talking about their enthusiasm for little computers, their nostalgia for the 1980s, what they thought ought to go into a small computer, what they thought ought to go into the educational side. So it was very lively,' said Liz.

As the forums filled with suggestions for what should be in the Pi, Liz's job was also to manage expectations: 'A lot of work was done explaining to people what the realities were, and what we could actually fit into the product if we were going to keep it at the price that it needed to be.'

Meanwhile, Eben was working on turning the prototype Pi into something that could actually be put into the hands of children. That meant seeking out a manufacturer, and at first he tried to do a deal with British companies, but they showed little interest in producing an ultra-cheap device. 'They gave you prices which were high either because their cost structure was rubbish or because they wanted you to go away. It's more polite to give you a useless price than it is just to say no.'

So inevitably that meant going to a Chinese company in Shenzhen, which over the space of 30 years had been transformed from a fishing village into the world capital of technology manufacturing, making just about everything from Apple's iPhone to washing machines and televisions. By the end of 2011 the Foundation had placed an order for 2,000 units. The plan now was to begin selling the Raspberry Pi on 29 February 2012. Eben had sent $50,000-worth of chips plus $50,000 in cash to Shenzhen – 'and then we waited and waited. November went past and December, then January and into February. And then one day ten samples turned up.'

The finished product was a little bigger than the version I had seen the previous year. It was now the size of a credit card rather than a USB stick, but remained a barebones device, looking like a component you might find inside a computer rather than a computer itself. And that initial plan for a price of £15 had collided with reality, and the device would retail at $35 or around £30.

But that did not dampen the excitement of those crowding onto the Raspberry Pi website for news. A post in early January announced that manufacturing had begun, explaining that while the team would have preferred to have the Pi made in Britain, they had reluctantly gone to China because UK businesses had offered a three-month schedule for manufacturing, compared to a three-to-four-week turnaround in the Far East. In early February a magazine interview with David Braben sparked a panic that consumers would not be able to get their hands on the Pi for six months, an idea Liz was quick to squash: 'You will be able to buy a Raspberry Pi from the end of February from this website.'

As the month progressed, the PR effort accelerated, even as the tension mounted about the timetable. In the days running up to 29 February I was taken to a school in Cambridge to film children getting to know the device, and I was lent one which we would have in the BBC News studio on launch day. What I did not realize at the time was that these were two of the precious ten machines that had so far arrived from China.

Behind the scenes, frantic efforts were going on to sign deals which would prove to be crucial to the project's success. As well as they had done to date, Upton, Braben, Jack Lang, Pete Lomas and the rest of the small team recognized that they did not have the skills or the resources to oversee a manufacturing and distribution effort on even a moderate scale. So they entered talks with two UK electronics component distributors, RS and Farnell. 'The thing I'm proudest of', says Eben Upton, 'was realizing that we had to become a licensing business, because there was no way we could supply the capital to scale.' The negotiations went right up to the wire. 'Farnell signed at six p.m. on the 28th of February. RS signed at two a.m. on the 29th.'

Two days earlier the Raspberry Pi blog had a post by Eben with the title, 'Ladies and gentlemen, set your alarms': 'The Raspberry Pi Foundation will be making a big (and very positive) announcement that *just might interest you* at 0600h GMT on Wednesday 29 February 2012. Come to www.raspberrypi.org to find out what's going on.' The 550 comments beneath showed the level of anticipation, and on that morning of the 29th a tidal wave of visitors swept first onto the

Raspberry Pi website and then onto the two much more robust sites of RS and Farnell, where you could actually order a Pi.

But very quickly, the two suppliers' websites crashed under the sheer weight of traffic from people desperate to get their hands on the device. Even the most optimistic forecast from one of the licensing firms had been that they might eventually sell 10,000 to 20,000 units. But by the end of the day something like 100,000 Raspberry Pis had been ordered. Remember, at this stage they had only ordered 2,000 from Shenzhen and even those had not arrived. 'We sold out of much more than what we didn't have,' says Eben Upton. 'We didn't just sell out the two thousand we didn't have: we sold *a hundred thousand*! Absolute cowboys!'

It was a few weeks later in March that a crate containing the first 2,000 arrived and was stored in Jack Lang's garage. 'I took one out of the top box,' says Eben, 'and we plugged it into his TV and it worked. Then we went down to the bottom of the pallet and took one out of a box at the bottom and that one worked as well. That's when we knew it was going to work.'

And by now it was all the more clear that they had been right to do the licensing deals. 'When you start talking hundreds of thousands or even millions of units, you're talking quite a big operation,' says David Braben with some understatement. 'It's not the sort of thing you can package by hand.' With the resources of Farnell and RS behind them, they could tell the Chinese manufacturer to ramp up production, although the last person to order on the opening day did not get their Raspberry Pi until four or five months later.

But over those months momentum continued to build. The tiny computer, whose creators originally had ambitions to make maybe 10,000 or 15,000 units for British schools, was rapidly becoming a global phenomenon. On the launch day, when the Raspberry Pi featured across BBC output at home and abroad, I had described it as 'a device which seems designed to make men of a certain age who cut their computing teeth as teenagers on a BBC Micro or a ZX Spectrum go all misty-eyed.' I also pointed out that 'some of them turned angry this morning as it became clear that they would not be getting their hands on the Raspberry Pi in a hurry.' Liz Upton says that amidst all the chaos most people were understanding 'but you still got people who were very, very angry about it – surprisingly for something that costs so little. But people were very invested in it.'

And at first that seemed to illustrate a problem for a project aimed at teenagers – interest was huge, but largely among middle-aged hobbyists rather than children. The community around it was extremely vibrant, with fans quickly building all sorts of Pi-related projects, but the tech-savvy contributors to the forums could be impatient towards those with less computing knowledge.

I first got my hands on one to test at home in April that year. As someone who had left school without ever touching a computer, I found it somewhat intimidating. Getting it working involved hunting down a spare keyboard and mouse and plugging it into the living-room TV, something which was not going to be popular in the homes of some teenagers. Fortunately, I had recruited 18-year-old coder Isabell Long to help me review the Pi, and she proved adept at getting it up and running. In a blogpost I described, with somewhat naive wonder, what happened next. 'Isabell opened a Python window and tried out a line of code. She typed in >>> print "Hello!", pressed return, and, lo and behold, the computer said "hello" back. One small step for coding...'

But what struck both me and Isabell was that it was not obvious how the barebones computer would instantly be welcomed in the classroom. 'Its components being so visible could put kids off,' she wrote. 'They're consumers, not programmers, at the moment, so seeing the electronics involved in what they use will either make them gasp in awe, or shy away in confusion or fear.' Getting the Raspberry Pi into classrooms did indeed prove to be quite a slow business, and would often depend on one enthusiastic teacher willing to set up an after-school club. For many state schools, and in particular their head teachers, the device just did not fit into a packed curriculum, especially while ICT was still the main computing GCSE.

But along with the middle-aged hobbyists, there were some teenage fans. Ryan Walmsley was 15 and studying for a slightly more specialized IT diploma when a teacher at his school in Cambridgeshire told him about the Pi. 'To think I could buy an entire computer for £30 was amazing, and the fact I could then take it to school with me to show off was great.' He tried to order one at 6 a.m. on launch day. 'I managed to finally get an order through while I was on the bus via my phone, and it arrived around four months later.' It changed his life. He became an active member of Liz Upton's online community starting various projects, he launched his own business selling Raspberry Pi accessories, and ended up working for a company which specialized in Pi products. At an event called Raspberry Jam a few months after the launch I met another young enthusiast. Eighteen-year-old Liam Fraser had set up a YouTube channel offering Raspberry Pi tutorials, and it had already had over a million views. A few years later, he got a job as an engineer with the charity.

But Ryan and Liam were exceptions. Most of the growing army of fans were adults, and they fuelled what felt like a rocket-powered take-off in the project which left the small team behind it gasping for breath. Eben Upton was still holding down his day job as a chip architect at Broadcom while overseeing the runaway train that was Raspberry Pi; Liz was overseeing the ever more demanding task of running the community and a communications team that was getting calls from around the world. 'We gave our lives to it,' Eben remembers. 'It was a really hard year.' There were huge challenges, such as waking up to the fact that the device needed CE marking, the European safety certification without which it could not be sold to consumers, let alone end up in schools.

But somehow they got through. Sales continued to surge, not just to individuals but to manufacturing companies that were finding a use for a cheap computing device in all sorts of industrial processes. Soon, accessories began to appear: some, like the camera module, built by Raspberry Pi, others, such as cases to make the barebones computer less intimidating, developed by external businesses. But the big development was that by September manufacturing had come home. At Pencoed in South Wales, Sony had a plant turning out high-end broadcast cameras, the opposite end of the pricing spectrum from the Raspberry Pi. After seeing BBC coverage of the launch, the plant's manager, David Jones, got in touch with Eben Upton to see if Sony could get involved.

At first neither of them thought it would be possible to make the sums add up and produce the Pi at a price to compete with what was on offer in Shenzhen. But then they thought about the cost of delivering from China, of having someone based there to oversee manufacturing, and the quality control issues the project was already encountering. With some investment by Sony in machinery which automated a key part of the process, they decided it could work, and within a couple of months British Pi production was up and running. Some manufacturing continued in China, but when I visited the Sony factory in October 2013, they were celebrating an amazing milestone: their one-millionth Raspberry Pi had just come off the production line. We filmed a process that appeared to be almost entirely automated, with only the assembly of the final components and then testing involving humans.

By this stage the Raspberry Pi had already far outstripped its creators' original ambitions. It had outsold the BBC Micro, and would eventually surge past the ZX Spectrum to become the bestselling British computer of all time.

In 2015, a new, even more basic model, the Raspberry Pi Zero, was launched with a £4 price tag, so cheap that it became the first computer to be given away with a magazine. Thousands rushed to get hold of a copy of *The Magpi*, a publication owned by Raspberry Pi Trading, which was expanding fast. In 2017, as the Sony plant celebrated production of its 10-millionth Raspberry Pi, Eben Upton told a Welsh business news site why it was important to build the device at home. 'We are particularly delighted that the Pi has set the benchmark for utilizing innovative and progressive manufacturing right here in the UK, as it was always our wish to make the computers in this country.'

But hold on a minute. What about the original mission? Back in 2011 when they first came to see me, Eben and David Braben had not talked about making a bestselling computer that would be exported around the world or proving that you could manufacture in the UK. Their idea had been all about changing the way children in the UK school system learned to interact with computers in the smartphone age, when they had vast computing power at their fingertips but no ability to look under the bonnet and see how things worked.

At first, there was a real danger that this mission would be knocked off course by the focus on commercial success. For some years I was a judge in an annual competition seeking the best Raspberry Pi projects in schools. In the first years, most of the entries were from private schools. The children showed off their Pi-powered weather stations or automated plant-watering schemes under the watchful eye of computing teachers who, one suspected, had played a key role in directing the projects. There was little evidence at first that many children in state schools were getting their hands on the Pi. Eben Upton admits that in the early stages that was a worry, but David Braben insists it was never the plan to get the Pi straight to children, because it was not ready for them. 'I was afraid we would almost mis-sell it into children's hands before it was ready to go,' he explains. 'It wasn't very turnkey: you needed to download things off the internet, you needed to be able to transfer them onto an SD card.'

What changed things was the realization that the project needed to be split into two arms, each with a clear direction. Raspberry Pi Trading, run by Eben, ran the commercial side, and an R&D division came up with new models and even began to look at developing its own chips. All of the trading profits went to the Raspberry Pi Foundation, a charity run by a former teacher, Philip Colligan, and charged with carrying out that original mission. This went on to merge with another educational initiative, Code Club, and was then selected by the UK government to run a National Centre for Computing Education with £82 million of public money.

Meanwhile, the argument that the way computing was taught in schools needed radical change had been won – but not necessarily with a good outcome for an economy increasingly short of the skills needed for the UK to prosper in the smartphone era. ICT had been phased out of the curriculum in English schools, replaced at GCSE and A-Level by the far more challenging Computer Science. Hurrah, said the likes of David Braben; about time too. But then the figures for exam entries came out.

By 2019 there had been a steep fall in the number of 16-year-olds getting some kind of computing qualification. However poor a subject ICT may have been – and there were now some teachers saying it had been unfairly maligned – large numbers of students took it, around 40 per cent of them girls. But a lack of trained teachers meant quite a lot of schools did not even offer Computer Science GCSE, and in any case its reputation as a subject in which it was much harder to get a good grade was off-putting both to pupils and to head teachers worried about slipping down league tables. As for diversity, in 2019 just 20 per cent of Computer Science GCSE entrants were girls. A report from Roehampton University found that between 2012 and 2017 the number of hours of computing taught in English secondary school classrooms had fallen by 31 per cent. There was growing concern that, while the UK might be doing better at bringing on star computer scientists, it was doing little to prepare the mass of the population for the digital age. One of the report's authors, Peter Kemp, put it like this: 'If the choice was to train Olympic champions or fight obesity, current computing provision appears to have picked the Olympians over the good health of the population, when we need both.'

But you could hardly blame Raspberry Pi for the government's failure to make the new computing curriculum work. It was the Pi community which was often to be found setting up code clubs in schools, and now the Foundation's skills were to be employed in finding and training the teachers needed to close the gap in computing education.

Late in 2019, I went to see Eben Upton at the Raspberry Pi Trading office on a Cambridge science park. The neighbours included the fast-growing cybersecurity firm Darktrace and a sadly empty space recently vacated by a games firm which had run out of money. Seventy staff – software developers, marketers, engineers – worked quietly here, and more than 130 across Cambridge at the offices of the Foundation. Eben took me into the R&D lab, picking up pieces of kit and swearing me to secrecy about one of the more ambitious projects. Then we sat and reflected on how far the project had come. If the original aim had been to increase the numbers applying to study Computer Science at Cambridge, it was job done: 'We have twice as many applying as we had at the height of the dot.com boom,' he said. 'And I understand from people that are still involved in the admissions process that, when you ask them, how did you get into computers, they say Raspberry Pi. Either because it's true, or because they've got the wit to pretend that they got involved.'

Just a few hundred metres away was the headquarters of the chip designer Arm, undoubtedly the most innovative tech firm to have been born in the UK over the last 30 years, and one whose history was inextricably bound up with that of Raspberry Pi.

Arm had been spun out of the BBC Micro manufacturer Acorn by, among others, Hermann Hauser, an Austrian-born scientist and entrepreneur who became a key figure in Cambridge's growth into a global player as a technology hub. At one stage Apple had owned 43 per cent of the business, and Hauser says the sale of that stake at a loss was what saved the ailing Californian company from going bust in the late 1990s.

By the time the iPhone came along, Arm's chip design was already becoming standard on mobile phones, and it quickly became the dominant force. 'We became the Intel of the mobile system,' says Hauser. So naturally the Raspberry Pi team came for advice to the man behind both the BBC Micro, whose success they were hoping to emulate, and the Arm chip which they were putting at the heart of their device. He laughs as he remembers what he told them: 'First of all, Raspberry Pi is a stupid name. And second, nobody's going to buy a bare circuit product – you've got to find a nice case and make it into a consumer product. They ignored both.' And of course he now accepts they were right, and that Raspberry Pi is a remarkable achievement for Cambridge and for the wider UK technology scene.

For Eben Upton that says something about the UK's potential as a tech nation. 'The Raspberry Pi experience shows there's an enormous amount of talent in the UK. And I think if you try and build a business, which stays focused on doing one thing, and doing it well, and you plug away at it year after year after year, you can build something that grows.' Despite starting with distinctly local aims, he insists it was important to think globally – rather than just about Britain.

> I'd much rather describe Raspberry Pi as being the third most popular general-purpose computing platform in the world than the most popular general-purpose computing platform in the UK. It's really important to us to have that kind of global ambition. I think we've got the talent here in the UK to make a go of it.

It may be tiny in comparison to Arm, with revenues of around £27 million in 2018 compared to the chip designer's £1.3 billion, but Raspberry Pi is still a British-run project. In 2016 Arm was bought by the Japanese technology investor SoftBank for $32 billion, around £24 billion. For Hermann Hauser, this was a tragedy, even if the deal was to prove extremely lucrative for him and other Arm shareholders. He told the BBC it was 'a sad day for technology in Britain', losing a company that was 'going to be used in all the next-generation phones and – more importantly – in the next generation of the internet of things'.

But four years later SoftBank, under pressure after a number of its extravagant bets on businesses such as the shared office space firm WeWork went wrong, decided to cash in. It sold Arm to Nvidia, the American company which had overtaken Intel to become the world's most valuable chipmaker, for $40 billion – a tidy profit, especially when you consider that the 2016 price had been seen as extremely generous.

If Hermann Hauser had been sad when Arm was first sold, this time he was incandescent. Despite his misgivings, he felt that SoftBank had been a good owner, keeping its promises to boost jobs and investment in Cambridge. In an open letter to the Prime Minister he warned that being owned by Nvidia would destroy an Arm business model that depended on being seen as a neutral supplier of designs by hundreds of chipmaker customers. What's more, if it was controlled by an American company the Cambridge business would now be subject to the whims of a US administration engaged in a bitter trade war with China, one of its key markets. 'Surrendering the UK's most powerful trade weapon to the US is making Britain a US vassal state,' he thundered, and called for the sale to be blocked. The trouble was, it was too late. The time for government intervention had been in 2016, but the sale to SoftBank soon after the EU referendum had been greeted by Theresa May's government as a vote of confidence in Brexit Britain.

From the 1980s on Cambridge had sought to paint itself as Silicon Fen, a hi-tech city where ideas from some of the world's leading scientists would emerge from the university's labs to form the basis of world-beating companies. For many years there was more hype than substance to this claim, but by the first decade of the twenty-first century billion-dollar businesses were thriving in Cambridge – not just Arm, but Cambridge Silicon Radio (CSR), and the data analysis firm Autonomy.

All three ended up in foreign hands: CSR sold to the American chipmaker Qualcomm, Autonomy to the American computer giant HP – which promptly wrote off most of the cost of its purchase a year later. Cambridge and the rest of the UK tech industry was by now proving itself adept at creating businesses that could thrive in the smartphone era, but less good at holding on to them once their backers sought a profitable exit.

As the Raspberry Pi story shows, the UK has plenty of talented engineers and entrepreneurs who are fizzing with ideas. In important areas of technology, from 5G to chip design to quantum computing, cutting-edge research is taking place in commercial laboratories and at some of the world's finest universities. Those universities and the opportunities to work in London's thriving tech sector have attracted talent from around the world. But, while the availability of capital for those starting and growing technology businesses has improved – and is certainly better than across the rest of Europe – there is still a short-term approach from the UK's finance industry which makes it hard to build world-beating companies.

Coupled with that is an attitude that has persisted for 30 years under both Labour and Conservative governments, that who owns a company does not really matter and should be decided by the market. Gone are the days when governments pick winners, and ministers can only intervene in a takeover when it is clear there are national security issues at stake.

There were, however, signs in 2020 that this might be changing. Boris Johnson's adviser Dominic Cummings arrived in Downing Street impatient to shake everything up and seeing Brexit as an opportunity to overturn what he saw as a 'this-is-how-we've-always-done-things' mindset in Whitehall – and that included industrial policy. He was an admirer of ARPA, the US government research agency that had been instrumental in sparking innovations from the internet to GPS, and was set on establishing something similar in the UK.

First evidence of this new activism came with the move by the government to splash out $500 million on a controlling stake in OneWeb, a failed venture to put 650 small satellites into low-level orbit as a means of providing a global broadband internet service. There was vague talk that it might also be used to give the UK its own independent form of GPS navigation – an American invention – after it became clear that Brexit meant an end to participation in the EU's Galileo project, which was trying to achieve the same thing.

It was clear the Civil Service did not think much of the whole idea of spending taxpayers' money on such a risky venture. The acting Permanent Secretary put on record her concern that all of the money could be lost – a move meant to signal, 'On your head be it . . .' But Cummings was not to be deterred, nor was he alone in thinking that the UK needed to have a stake in the technologies of the future rather than just sit back and watch the United States and China dominate them.

Key to that concern was the field of artificial intelligence, another area where the UK had lots of brainpower but very little financial ownership. The rise of intelligent machines promised to change our lives even more radically than the smartphone. Or perhaps to kill us all . . .

5

The End of the Human Race?

In 2011, four years after the birth of the iPhone and the dawn of the social smartphone era, we were becoming used to owning devices which appeared to do just about everything. We used them to summon a cab, to order our shopping or to check the football scores or weather. Runners and cyclists relied on them to monitor their performance and, for just about anyone under 30, a smartphone app was where they went to hook up with a new partner.

And in 2011, Apple unveiled Siri, and we started to get used to talking to our phones and having them answer us back. In a demo at the launch of the iPhone 4S, an Apple executive put the voice assistant through its paces, asking it whether he needed a raincoat and getting the response, 'It sure looks like rain today.'

At first Siri did not get much attention, perhaps because the death of Apple's founder Steve Jobs was announced a couple of days later. But this was the start of a trend that would see smart voice-controlled assistants become a common feature of all kinds of devices from Android phones to Amazon's Echo smart speaker.

And this all signalled that another powerful new wave of technology was arriving with the promise of an even more profound impact on the economy and society than the smartphone or social media. Because what lay behind the smart assistants was a sudden rapid advance in two artificial intelligence technologies: speech recognition and natural language processing.

Companies like Apple and Google, Microsoft and Amazon had begun investing large sums in research into artificial intelligence, buying start-up companies in the field and hiring leading academic experts. But for most smartphone users AI was still science fiction. They were almost certainly unaware that behind everything from Amazon recommendations to the way their phones sorted through their photos and recognised the different faces of their friends lay a great leap forward in techniques such as machine learning. The first *Terminator* film had been released in 1984, Steven Spielberg's *AI* had come out in 2001, but nobody was looking at Siri or the Google Assistant and thinking that robots were about to take over. Until December 2014.

That was when my interview with Stephen Hawking sparked a global debate about the existential threat posed by artificial intelligence. In the autumn of that year a public relations executive at the chipmaker Intel contacted me to see if I was interested in an interview with the man who was undoubtedly Britain's most famous scientist. For more than 40 years the physicist Stephen Hawking had been paralysed and confined to a wheelchair as a result of motor neurone disease. The condition had been expected to kill him within a few years, but he defied expectations and, while his body was increasingly useless, his mind remained as sharp as ever. His work as a scientist continued, his fame grew with the publication of his internationally bestselling book *A Brief History of Time*, but all the while he was dependent on technology to keep him alive and enable him to communicate.

At the centre of the communications system was quite an ancient Windows PC, controlled by a sensor activated by a muscle in his cheek. This allowed the professor to type emails and other documents or have his words spoken by that robotic Hawking voice which had become so familiar. Now that technology was getting an overhaul from a consortium of companies led by Intel.

The new system included an element of artificial intelligence, in the form of predictive text technology, which would speed up Hawking's laborious writing process by learning his style and anticipating what he would say next.

This had been produced by a Cambridge company called SwiftKey, one of Britain's most successful AI start-ups, which had built a popular predictive text keyboard for smartphones. It was soon to be bought by Microsoft.

Artificial intelligence research has gone in cycles, with periods of despondency known as AI winters when scientists appeared to have hit a dead end. In the 1990s and the early years of the twenty-first century there had been just such a period, when divisions between researchers over which path to take in the quest to build intelligent machines and a lack of big breakthroughs had seen funding slow to a trickle. But for the last few years there had been a sense that spring was coming. Dozens of fledgling tech firms were emerging to advance the field, and many of the most promising AI scientists were based in the UK.

I was of course delighted to get this rare opportunity to interview Stephen Hawking, even if Intel clearly hoped this would be an opportunity to promote its innovations. But an encounter with the scientist had to be carefully prepared weeks in advance. Even with his new technology you could not just sit down in front of a TV camera for an off-the-cuff to-and-fro. Instead, you had to send off your questions by email and await his replies, and then, at some stage after that, you would meet to record what was effectively a scripted conversation. I thought hard about the half-dozen questions which might yield something interesting and newsworthy.

I asked what difference his new system would make to the way he worked, why he had chosen to retain his old computer voice rather than get a much more human version as the technology would have allowed, and threw in a few wider questions about how the internet had changed his life and whether he saw it as a force for good.

Then I ended with this: 'When you watch software engineers and machine learning experts at work as they have been on this project, how far along the path to artificial intelligence do you think we are?'

I sent my questions off via the Intel PR person and waited. A couple of weeks later I was told that the professor had been taken ill, and both his answers and our filming would have to be postponed. Then finally, around four weeks later, an email arrived with the replies to my questions. As I scanned them they all seemed fine, if not particularly revelatory, though his character shone through.

With his old system, he said, he had written five books, 'including *A Brief History of Time*, which was on the *Sunday Times* bestseller list for over five years, longer than any other book. The Bible and Shakespeare don't count, apparently.' He hadn't wanted a new voice because his old one had become his trademark, 'and I'm told that children who need a computer voice, want one like mine.'

Then I landed on the last question, the one about AI – and gulped at his response:

> The primitive forms of artificial intelligence we already have, have proved very useful. But I think the development of full artificial intelligence could spell the end of the human race. Once humans develop artificial intelligence, it would take off on its own, and re-design itself at an ever-increasing rate. Humans, who are limited by slow biological evolution, couldn't compete, and would be superseded.

Now, this was a story and a very good one the world's most famous scientist says AI will make humans obsolete. The only problem was that everything depended on him actually saying it, and Hawking's health appeared to be fragile.

Nevertheless, a few weeks later we were at the Savoy Hotel, where the scientist was due to attend a press conference to unveil his new system. We were shown into rather a grand room where Hawking and his team were waiting.

Confronted with this extraordinary human being, my crew and I were at first a little awkward. Communication with someone whose only way of interacting with others was by twitching a muscle in his cheek appeared challenging. But everybody got on with their job, setting up one camera trained on him, another on me, testing microphones and adjusting the lighting.

Then there was a hitch. Hawking's team was struggling with the computer which would read out his answers to my questions. They fiddled around, increasingly exasperated – and then resorted to the time-honoured trick for fixing recalcitrant technology. They turned it off and on again. The computer came back to life and we were ready to go. I asked my scripted questions, and Hawking's machine generated the answers we knew were coming, including that crucial final one about AI's threat to the human race.

We finished, packed up and all had our photo taken with the great man, then returned to New Broadcasting House to slice and dice our story in many different versions for the BBC's many different outlets. My key task was to make a TV package for the flagship *Six O'Clock* and *Ten O'Clock News* bulletins, which featured, inevitably, a clip of the movie *Terminator* to illustrate Hawking's nightmarish vision of AI bringing an end to the human race. But there was also an interview with the leading artificial intelligence scientist Professor Murray Shanahan of Imperial College, who gave us a more measured view of the technology's potential for good as well as harm. I wrote a long news story for the BBC News website, which contained a video featuring the whole conversation with Stephen Hawking and another clip in which Professor Shanahan provided a beginner's guide to AI.

Interest was huge – many millions read the online story, and Hawking's warning became news right around the world. He joined the likes of the tech entrepreneur Elon Musk, who had called AI 'our biggest existential threat', in triggering a debate about where this field of research was taking us. What was striking to me at the time was that a man who was seeing his life augmented by a computer, and the workings of his brain beginning to be mirrored in SwiftKey's software, should be so concerned about where all this was heading.

Many of those who were intimately involved in this research were exasperated by what they saw as headline-grabbing alarmism:

'I was gobsmacked, astonished,' remembers Professor Michael Wooldridge, who was leading AI research at Oxford University. 'I was looking around at my colleagues and thinking, who's going to respond to that? Who's going to stand up and say bluntly, you're worrying about the wrong thing?'

But another computer scientist, Southampton University's Professor Wendy Hall, was not sure that the warning was out of place. Professor Hall, a close collaborator with the creator of the Web, Tim Berners-Lee, was later to be asked to chair a government review on growing AI in the UK. 'He was right,' she says. 'If we can develop artificial general intelligence then, potentially, the machines will evolve faster than us. And we will end up being the slaves to the machine, as opposed to the other way around.'

And the news story did serve a purpose. As well as forcing the scientists to come out of their labs and start thinking about and debating the implications of their work, it alerted the wider public to the fact that a new and exciting technology could be about to change their lives. They were just getting used to the smartphone and social media revolution, but now the massive amounts of data that people were creating and sharing using these new tools was fuelling a new wave of technological change.

Because by 2014, an AI boom was under way, and London was one of its epicentres. In January that year a company called DeepMind, that appeared to have no products and negligible revenues, was acquired by Google for the unlikely sum of £400 million.

DeepMind had been founded in 2010 by an extraordinary young polymath, Demis Hassabis, and two friends, Mustafa Suleyman and Shane Legg. Hassabis, born in London to parents he describes as technophobes, was a child prodigy, mastering chess at five, going on to be the second-best player in the world for his age group at 13, and passing his A-levels at 15. Like Eben Upton and David Braben, he combined an academic career which saw him study at Cambridge and then University College London with a fascination for video games, which proved both profitable and intellectually stimulating.

He was still a teenager when he got a job with the games developer Bullfrog, and was one of the creators of Theme Park, a hugely successful title which sold more than 15 million copies worldwide. The game is a simulation where players try to build profitable theme parks, success being dependent on how visitors react to the world that you create for them. In effect, it is a sandpit for experimenting with ever more complex systems that try to emulate human behaviour. Games development might sound a trivial activity, but for Demis Hassabis and others it has proved a fertile training ground in the quest to understand human intelligence and then try to replicate it in computers.

One evening Hassabis's boss at Bullfrog, Peter Molyneux, took him along to a board games group run by Ian Livingstone, a fantasy writer who had become a big figure in the video games industry as the creative chief at Eidos, publisher of Tomb Raider. Livingstone instantly took to the young developer – 'He had huge charisma, was very confident and super-bright, and loved playing board games as well as video games. Not only bright but charming.' Remembering that evening, which was to mark the beginning of a long friendship, the veteran games entrepreneur told me how delighted he had been to beat the young Hassabis and the others in the group at a board game called Africa. 'I double-crossed everyone with a horrendous back-stabbing move – I think it was a lesson in life for him!'

In 2020, sitting at a table in his corner office at DeepMind headquarters, with a fine view over the London skyline, Demis Hassabis grinned when I brought this up. 'Ian reminds me of that every time I see him.' But looking back more than 20 years, he was clear about the wider lessons he'd been taught by all kinds of games. 'All the games I wrote had AI in them, with characters or creatures all with AI under the hood, that you interacted with as the player, so they were all simulation games.' When he started his own games company, Elixir Studios, it was once again to build a simulation, Republic: The Revolution.

Ian Livingstone signed the game up for Eidos: 'It was a very ambitious project, a living, breathing city, and everybody you met you could interact with and learn from. You had to try and get control of the media and the government.' Livingstone says the game was ahead of its time, built to run on hardware that did not exist back then. It was a failure, but Hassabis said it was probably for the best: 'Maybe it was a blessing in disguise. It gave me a chance to re-think about AI and stuff that I'd been thinking about since I was a teenager and just sort of figuring out, was it the right time to get back into that?'

Meanwhile, he was adding another element to the range of skills he would need to fulfil that teenage dream of advancing artificial intelligence. Working on a neuroscience doctorate at University College London, he found himself at the forefront of the new wave of AI thinking:

> I got a lot of information about how the brain works. I did some work myself on memory and imagination – really interesting processes that the brain does that we don't know how to do in computers. And so I felt that I had quite a unique take on what was happening.

It is worth pausing here to remember just how far out of fashion AI had gone in the late 1990s.

In the last 30 years of the twentieth century the discipline had been riven by deep divisions. One camp, led by the British academic Geoff Hinton, believed the way forward lay with neural networks, essentially software that mimicked the way the brain works. The other approach, symbolic AI, involved modelling the mind and its cognitive processes, such as how we solve problems and think in sentences. You could sum it up as the neural network crowd trying to build a brain, with thousands of nodes across which data flows, whereas the symbolic AI types were trying to gain a deeper understanding of how we think.

In the late 1980s the AI mainstream decided that neural networks were not the way forward, and Geoff Hinton moved to Canada in search of funding. 'They went out of fashion,' says Professor

Michael Wooldridge, 'for the simple reason that the processors weren't fast enough to be able to cope with the algorithms that people developed.'

But in the first decade of the twenty-first century neural networks came roaring back, along with a branch of AI called machine learning, where a computer learns to complete a task without being given explicit instructions after being trained with labelled data. For instance, it might be fed thousands of scans showing brain tumours, with each labelled as either malignant or benign, so that it could learn to differentiate between them. 'What happened was we got more processing power,' says Wendy Hall. 'And partly through the use of internet and social media, we got a lot more data, and that came together to create the big AI hype that we have now.' The accelerating ownership of smartphones also provided rocket fuel for the AI boom, says Michael Wooldridge. 'They gave us all a camera that was connected to the internet, they gave us all a typewriter that was connected to the internet, and all of a sudden there was just this huge new source of data available.'

Demis Hassabis had studied computer science in the 1990s at Cambridge, where symbolic AI was very much in vogue, but had then watched the latest developments in neural networks and machine learning. He knew which side he was on.

> If I told you, can you type out a bunch of rules for how you swim, or how you ride a bike, that's very difficult, because you're doing it intuitively with your motor cortex, and that kind of intuition and pattern-matching, which humans do really well with our brains, symbolic systems are terrible at. And of course that's what deep learning and reinforcement learning and the new neural network learning systems are very good at: mimicking a lot of this sort of intuitive capability and pattern-matching that we take for granted, as we do it effortlessly.

So by 2010, he had developed some understanding of how the brain worked, his work in games development had helped him think about how to simulate human interactions, and he had suffered his first failure as a businessman. Just about the perfect grounding then to start his own AI business.

All he and his friends Shane Legg and Mustafa Suleyman needed was a serious chunk of money from investors willing to fund blue-sky research that might not produce a payback for a decade. That was going to be impossible to find from conventional venture capitalists, with AI still provoking, in Demis's words, 'eye-rolling' even in academia. What was needed, he decided, was a billionaire with a passion for this area of science. Where might they be found? Obviously in Silicon Valley, but the three of them had no contacts out there. Then they found out about an event held in San Francisco by the Singularity University, an institution dedicated to the idea that the moment when artificial general intelligence arrives and humans are overtaken by machines is within reach. One of their target billionaires was going to be at the event.

Hassabis managed to get an invitation to speak, and his presentation, entitled 'A systems neuroscience approach to building AGI', laying out the big advances in understanding the brain and what they implied for artificial intelligence research, was well received. But that was not the point – he still needed to meet his billionaire. A cocktail reception at the conference would provide an opportunity, but he knew that the man in question would be besieged by supplicants just like him, and getting his attention would involve something special.

On an in-house podcast produced by DeepMind Hassabis tells the story of how, once again, a game came to his rescue. He had researched his target and found that they had a common passion for chess.

So I used my number-one fact on chess, which even surprises grandmasters, that, thinking about it from a games designer's point of view – why is chess such a great game? how did it evolve into such a great game? – my belief is that it is actually because of the creative tension between the bishop and the knight.

In his minute with the billionaire he explained that, while the bishop and knight were worth the same, their different powers produced a creative asymmetry that made chess a fascinating game. 'I don't know how I managed to crowbar that into a drinks party, but it made him stop and think, which is exactly what I was hoping.'

The next day Hassabis and his team were invited back to pitch their business idea, and this investor and a couple of others agreed to supply the few million dollars needed to get DeepMind started.

So who was the mystery billionaire? Demis Hassabis has never confirmed the name, but it is widely assumed to be Peter Thiel, the PayPal co-founder and Facebook investor who later became just about the only Silicon Valley figure close to Donald Trump. Even in 2020, when I said, 'Come on – it was Peter Thiel!' Hassabis laughed and said if I had got there by a process of triangulation, so be it, but he could not confirm it.

The funding meant they could start work, recruiting some brilliant people who back then, before the AI boom, were still relatively cheap to hire. They were confident that they had the right approach for what was a ridiculously ambitious goal. Their mission statement talked of 'solving intelligence', which sounds as though they thought they were charting a clear path to the artificial general intelligence which so frightened Stephen Hawking. But they still had to prove it. 'We were definitely at the front of the pack, but we were not sure it was going to work.'

It was three years before they became confident that they were onto something. Once again, it was to be games that provided the laboratory for their experiments, in this case very simple retro video games played on an Atari console, the likes of Pong and Space Invaders that you might have played on a pub machine in the 1980s. The point of the exercise was not to show that a computer could outperform a human at a game – after all, machines had already conquered much harder challenges, from chess to Scrabble. But a chess program could not go off and play Scrabble: what DeepMind hoped to develop was a system that could learn to play different games, and then perhaps undertake all sorts of other tasks. Beating

Pong, then, would be just one small step along the path to creating artificial general intelligence.

At first, Demis remembers, they seemed to be getting nowhere. 'I think it was three months, maybe six months, that we couldn't even win a point at Pong. And we're like, oh, well, maybe we'll never ever even do Pong.'

Even when they won their first point they thought it might be a fluke. Then, a month later, they won their first game, and soon they were beating the Pong system 21–0. They then moved on to the more complex challenge of Space Invaders, and eventually managed to achieve world record scores on this and five other Atari games.

In 2013 the Atari project led to DeepMind's first paper in the journal *Nature*, explaining the deep learning and reinforcement-learning techniques. The Atari agent had been given only minimal information about the games it was playing – effectively it was like an alien who had wandered into a pub and started playing Space Invaders without even knowing the rules.

Meanwhile, others were making rapid progress using similar techniques. In 2012 two students of Geoff Hinton entered the annual ImageNet competition, a test to see how accurately an AI system could identify objects within a vast database of photos. They trounced the opposition. It was becoming clear that if deep learning could allow a computer to see and interpret the world around it – understand, for instance, the difference between a dog and a cat – then all sorts of useful applications, from self driving cars to robot radiographers, would become possible.

Google promptly hired Hinton and his students to join its fast-growing and well-funded AI research. Late in 2013 the search giant made a more expensive acquisition, snapping up Boston Dynamics, which had made a name for itself with YouTube videos of its startlingly nimble and slightly alarming robots.

But when the deal which in January of 2014 saw the search giant pay $600 million to acquire DeepMind was announced, it came out of nowhere for both financial and technology specialists. 'Google makes its biggest EU purchase yet with the technology that aims to make computers think like humans,' read a *Guardian* headline. 'British chess prodigy sells artificial intelligence software firm to Google for £242 million,' said the *Daily Mail*.

At Oxford University, a man whose whole career had been all about artificial intelligence, was thinking, '. . . Who?' Professor Michael Wooldridge admits with some embarrassment that at that stage he and his colleagues in the Computer Science department had not even heard of DeepMind. 'We were astonished, I think, that this company that had no products, apparently no business plan, no customers, had been acquired for this astonishing sum of money.'

The deal also sparked questions about why the UK, where so much groundbreaking research in artificial intelligence was being done in university labs and in start-ups, could not provide the finance to keep fledgling businesses such as DeepMind and SwiftKey independent. Why had British banks and venture capitalists, or perhaps a British technology giant such as Vodafone or the aero engine-maker Rolls-Royce, not stepped in to keep such a promising asset under UK ownership?

Well, partly because they, like the AI academics, had probably never heard of DeepMind before it was swallowed by Google. Then again, that obscurity was all part of Demis Hassabis's grand plan. 'We didn't want the big companies realizing we were making the kind of progress we were making, and therefore ramping up their own AI efforts in competition with us. So for a while the idea was to stay under the radar.'

Now they were part of one of those big companies, although the founders insisted as part of the deal that they would stay in London. Suddenly the strategy switched, and DeepMind, perhaps to convince the new paymasters that they had spent wisely, came out of the shadows. Consciously or not, DeepMind became the poster child for the AI revolution and the benefits it could deliver. Within a couple of years the company and its scientists were making headlines around the world, and once again it was a game that provided the pathway to a new advance in AI.

In 1997 IBM's Deep Blue had defeated the chess world champion Gary Kasparov: a signal, it had seemed at the time, that machines would soon outpace humans in many complex intellectual pursuits. But the supercomputer had won by brute force, searching through millions of moves in seconds, rather than using creativity. The AI community decided that a much more challenging test would be the ancient Chinese game of Go. Apparently invented more than 2,500 years ago, the strategy game involves laying out black or white stones on a grid with the aim of encircling your opponent. It looks simple enough, but the beauty of the game is that the number of possible moves is vastly greater than in chess; indeed, it is said to be greater than the number of atoms in the universe. 'Go is the purest game in the world,' says Ian Livingstone. 'I can teach it you in thirty seconds, but it will take a lifetime to master.' That meant it would be impossible for a supercomputer to beat it by analysing every possible move, and AI experts predicted that human masters of Go would be safe from a challenge for many decades.

But one March day in 2016 I found myself asking a producer to pop out and buy a Go board. News had emerged that day that a master Go player, Lee Se-dol, was 3–0 down to a computer program in a best-of-five contest in Seoul in South Korea. The program was called AlphaGo, and it had been created by DeepMind. Demis Hassabis had first encountered Go while at Cambridge University, and, typically, had quickly become rather good at it, though he was certainly far from master level.

DeepMind's quest to master Go had been an exercise on a much more ambitious level than the small team taking on Space Invaders and Pong in a mission to 'solve intelligence', in terms of the science, the resources available under the Google banner, and the way the project was designed to burnish the image of DeepMind. AlphaGo used a combination of AI techniques to set about the task of beating Lee Se-dol. It was fed a database of historic games with more than 30 million moves to learn how humans play. Later, it played different versions of itself many millions of times to learn from its mistakes.

The match against Lee Se-dol was a major entertainment event across Asia, with Go pundits analysing each move and an audience of 200 million watching online. As the contest at Seoul's Four Seasons Hotel got under way, most AI experts and just about every Go aficionado expected the 18-times world champion to win with ease.

At first each game appeared to be a very tight and evenly matched contest, but on each occasion AlphaGo drew away at the end to win. In the second game, one of its moves proved hugely surprising to the commentators. 'That's a very strange move,' said one of the pundits, himself a master Go player. Another was convinced it was a rare mistake by the machine. So bamboozled was Lee Se-dol by move 37 in the game that he left the room for 15 minutes to clear his head. Afterwards he admitted that, whereas he had been taken by surprise by his defeat in the first game, he had been ill at ease throughout this second encounter. 'From the very beginning of the game I did not feel like there was a point that I was leading.'

David Silver, leader of the AlphaGo project, told *Wired* that the program had calculated that there was a one-in-10,000 chance that a human player would have made move 37, but it had looked back through the vast archive of games it had played against itself and forward to what might happen next, and played it anyway. 'It knows everything, and can play creatively,' one young South Korean Go player watching the contest told the *LA Times*. 'All but the very best Go players craft their style by imitating top players. AlphaGo seems to have totally original moves it creates itself.'

At a press conference after AlphaGo went 3–0 up, making victory inevitable, Demis Hassabis was gracious, praising the brilliance of Lee Se-dol. And in one last hurrah for humanity, the Korean player went on to win the fourth game, before the series ended 4–1 to the robot player. As if to emphasise how keen DeepMind was to emerge from the shadows, the story of AlphaGo was told in a Netflix documentary which had full access over many months to the team behind the project. The company then held a London premiere of the film, with Demis Hassabis and David Silver appearing on stage afterwards with the director to answer questions.

The Go project did not end there. Eighteen months later DeepMind unveiled AlphaGo Zero, a new program using a far leaner, lighter approach. Instead of being fed huge amounts of data from previous human games, it was simply given some basic information about the rules of Go, told to play against itself, and informed after each game whether it had won or lost. Within 72 hours it had become so expert that it beat AlphaGo – the human-trained version which had defeated Lee Se-dol – by 100 games to nil, and within 40 days had overtaken all the subsequent versions of the program. This success meant another paper in *Nature*, and another press conference where David Silver explained why this mattered. 'It shows it's the novel algorithms that count, not the compute power or the data.' This seemed to contradict the accepted wisdom that it was advances in computing that were driving progress in AI – instead, it appeared it was the sheer brain power of the DeepMind engineers designing those algorithms that was decisive.

Silver also enthused about an idea that I described at the time as rather scary – that in just a few days a machine had surpassed the knowledge of this game acquired by humanity over thousands of years: 'We've actually removed the constraints of human knowledge, and it's able, therefore, to create knowledge itself from first principles, from a blank slate.' DeepMind then took this lean data approach, renamed it AlphaZero, and showed that it could work for other games, notably chess

But for all its mastery of games, for all the showmanship, the company has continued to face two nagging questions: what are the practical uses of its technology? And will it end up harming us?

It has certainly cost Google a lot of money. The DeepMind team now occupies one floor in Google's St Pancras offices, and has spilled over into another nearby building. Accounts filed at Companies House showed that in 2018 it made a loss of $570 million, up from $341 million the year before. The reason: hiring more and more of the most brilliant minds in AI – people who had been relatively cheap in 2010 but now commanded six-figure starting salaries. Meanwhile, the revenues its work provided to the parent company, now renamed Alphabet, remained negligible.

Demis Hassabis insists that his team has delivered and will continue to deliver tangible results both for its American paymasters and for humanity as a whole. He points to a machine learning project to cut energy use in data centres by as much as 20 per cent, potentially saving Google huge sums, though there have been some questions about whether a wider trend to more energy-efficient techniques can be credited solely to DeepMind. He insists a whole range of big meaty problems, from climate change to the discovery of new drugs, will be addressed by his team over the next decade. 'We've trained all our algorithms, and then we've beaten all the games that are out there. What I'm hoping you're going to see in the next phase of AI – especially for us – is some huge breakthroughs in Nobel Prize-level-winning problems.'

More immediately, DeepMind's work on using AI to triage scans of eyes has the potential to produce great benefits for the National Health Service and its patients, although much of this work has now been swallowed up by Google's Health division. But having emerged from obscurity to become the poster boy for AI, and an emblem of the UK's strength in this emerging technology, DeepMind has also been the focus for the growing debate about its ethical use.

At the premiere of the Netflix AlphaGo film, a member of the audience asked Demis Hassabis whether such a powerful technology needed to be regulated. He used a line he has employed frequently about any technology being neutral: it is just how we decide to use it that determines whether it is good or bad. And, having launched DeepMind back in 2010 at a conference dedicated to the idea that artificial general intelligence, with all its potential for machines to outpace humans and make them obsolete, was an imminent possibility, he seemed keen to downplay what had been achieved so far. 'It's still very early-stage,' he told the enthusiast for regulation.

We won at Go. But the real world is way more complex than even Go is, so there's a long way to go, even though we've made some impressive advances. That gives us the time in the research community to research all these deep questions about what are the right control mechanisms, what are the right ways to specify goals, and what are the limits of these systems.

Until that research had been done, he said, it was too early to start talking about regulation.

Plenty of people disagreed, pointing out that, long before the advent of killer robots, there were already lots of urgent ethical questions to be addressed. Suddenly everyone seemed to be boasting that they were using AI (they meant machine learning) to improve their processes: lawyers, insurance firms, town planners – even the police were getting in on the act.

But what if their algorithms – which in any case they did not understand – were baking in human biases: deciding that people from certain neighbourhoods should get a lower credit rating, or that someone from an ethnic minority should not be shortlisted for a job? Facial recognition was being deployed on the streets of London, but was it reliable, and did we want to live in a society where our biometric data was available in the cloud, for access by law enforcement or by companies wanting to track us and sell us more stuff? DeepMind and its Google parent quickly realised that these questions could not simply be put on the shelf for another day. They set up ethics panels, hired philosophers, sociologists – and hundreds of lobbyists – and tried to get ahead of the game.

We started this chapter with Stephen Hawking's nightmare vision of humans made redundant by the full AI that Demis Hassabis was pursuing, in a mission enthusiastically backed by Peter Thiel, a man who has bought a home in New Zealand, something once described as 'billionaire apocalypse insurance'.

I asked the DeepMind founder whether he had been exasperated by that pronouncement. He revealed that a few months later he had met Professor Hawking at his home in Cambridge.

He invited me up – actually we were supposed to spend an hour together, we ended up spending four or five hours. I remember his nurses coming in and trying to pull him out and getting his lunch and he was sort of saying no, I want to carry on talking.

The physicist, perhaps aware that this was an area of science where his visitor had far greater expertise, let him do most of the talking. 'He was really fascinated. He asked me a lot of probing questions about what we were building, what we were trying to do. And by the end of it he was very much more reassured.'

A couple of years after his doom-laden interview, and after that meeting with Demis Hassabis, Stephen Hawking made another intervention into the debate about AI. Speaking in Cambridge at an event marking the opening of the Centre for the Study of Intelligence, he gave an overview of where we had got to so far. He talked of the potential of the technology to eradicate disease and poverty, and combat climate change, while warning again of the danger of machines developing a will of their own, in conflict with humanity. But, he concluded, 'In short, the rise of powerful AI will be either the best, or the worst thing, ever to happen to humanity. We do not yet know which.' Hearing this speech, Demis Hassabis decided his meeting had made an impact. At least the great scientist was now open to the possibility that the AI adventure would not end in disaster.

6

Elon Musk and the Triumph of Tech

Think about life in 2007 and what you could not do then that is now second nature. If you wanted a taxi, you had to hail one on the street or walk to a cab rank. If you fancied a takeaway, you hunted through the kitchen drawer for the menu from the local Indian restaurant. Organizing a family or school reunion, and then sharing photos afterwards, meant an endless and complex chain of emails.

Getting off the train in a town you didn't know meant stopping a stranger and asking for directions, interacting with a human rather than a phone. Changing the temperature in the living room involved walking to the thermostat rather than adjusting it remotely via an app on the way home. To get the latest news about your sports team or hear a warning about bad weather you had to turn on the TV or radio or pick up a newspaper, rather than be alerted by those urgent pings from smartwatches and phones that have become a constant soundtrack in many offices and homes.

And if you were a prime minister or a president, conveying your thoughts to a grateful nation necessitated inviting in some grubby journalists who might get the wrong end of the stick. How much more simple and gratifying to knock out a tweet and speak directly, unfiltered, to the world.

So rapidly have these technologies – the smartphone, social media, AI – become woven into our lives that we have become blasé about them. But maybe we are right to be slightly underwhelmed. For these innovations, ingenious as they may seem, have in some ways been relatively trivial, making marginal rather than dramatic changes to the way we live. The entrepreneur Peter Thiel summed up this disappointed view of the smartphone era thus: 'We wanted flying cars, instead we got 140 characters.' He was referring of course to the original length of a tweet, now doubled to 280 characters, and looking back wistfully to mid-twentieth-century visions of the future.

I was born in 1958 and, two weeks after my birth in Queen Charlotte's Hospital in West London, the Americans launched their first satellite, playing catch-up with the Soviet Union, which had sent Sputnik into space the previous year. The space race was under way, and in 1961 President John F. Kennedy made his dramatic and surely unrealistic pledge to put an American on the Moon by the end of the decade.

But, sure enough, in 1969, a global audience of millions (not including me – my mum had sent me to bed after seeing Apollo 11 land) watched Neil Armstrong's 'one small step for man, one giant leap for mankind'. The Moon had been conquered, in the same amount of time that Apple took the iPhone from version 1 to the 6S, and surely all sorts of achievements would now follow, from lunar settlements to a mission to Mars. We were confident then of a future that would include, as well as space travel, homes full of robots, limitless energy, a 20-hour working week and – yes, flying cars.

The reality has of course been rather different. The smartphone era has been mostly about advances in software rather than hardware or infrastructure, which is perhaps why any impact on economic growth has been virtually impossible to detect. The 'weightless' parts of our economy – smartphone apps, e-commerce, video streaming – advanced at breakneck speed in the decades since the 1960s, while the heavy stuff – manufacturing, construction and, in particular, transport – lumbered along in the slow lane. Clogged-up roads meant motoring became slower and more polluting, air travel got slower with the retirement of Concorde, manned space travel went into retreat, and in the UK building a high-speed rail network was scheduled to take more than twice the time it took to deliver President Kennedy's lunar ambitions.

But in the twenty-first century one man has recaptured that 1960s optimism about what technology can achieve. He has set off on a mission to revive space travel, to transform motoring and to find cleaner sources of energy. His name is Elon Musk, and he has done more than anyone, perhaps even more than the father of the iPhone, Steve Jobs, to enthuse people about the potential of technology.

That, at least, was what I told my bosses at the BBC in the autumn of 2015. This was the time of year when I made my annual pitch for funding to go to CES, the January gadgetfest in Las Vegas. For me, it was an opportunity to tell mainstream audiences about technology trends that they might not hear about at other times of the year.

But, as budgets got tighter, selling CES became harder, as editors became more indifferent to each new marginal improvement in smartphones or home automation. What's the *big* theme this year? they would ask. If I told them the event would be all about AI they would shrug and say that was what I'd offered last year.

So that autumn I decided on a different approach. As well as heading for Las Vegas to cover CES, we would deliver an interview with the single most exciting person in tech, Elon Musk, at his base in California. Musk, I explained, a South African-born engineer and entrepreneur who had made his fortune as a co-founder of PayPal, was making huge audacious bets in a number of areas. His SpaceX business was set on revolutionizing space travel, and was pioneering the design of rockets that could deliver satellites into orbit and then return to Earth to be re-used. But that was just for starters. The company defined its ultimate goal as 'enabling people to live on other planets'. Another venture, Solar City, was on a mission to combat global warming by developing more efficient solar energy and producing batteries for energy storage. But the main focus of our interest was Tesla, the electric carmaker which was already making the old automotive giants sit up and wonder whether they might be facing obsolescence.

My pitch worked. The editors decided that an interview with Elon Musk sounded like a good idea, and we booked our flights to Las Vegas with a side trip to California to visit the Tesla factory in

Fremont. There was just one problem. By that point I had not actually confirmed our interview. I made my pitch to Tesla PR executives in both London and California, stressing that the interview would run across the BBC's output, reaching hundreds of millions of people around the world. They seemed moderately enthusiastic but stressed that, while a visit to the factory could certainly be arranged, an encounter with the mercurial tycoon could not be guaranteed.

So through November and December we waited. And waited. At the beginning of January I flew out to Las Vegas with my producer Jat Gill and cameraman Steve Adrain, who had filmed the iPhone launch with me eight years earlier. We ran around in our jet-lagged state getting footage of virtual reality headsets – VR was all the rage that year – robots, and plenty of car technology. But still we waited for news from Tesla.

Then finally the call came through. Elon Musk would see us – not at his Fremont factory, but at the Tesla Design Centre in Los Angeles. That meant extra costs – our flights home had been booked from San Francisco – but fortunately the powers that be back home were so relieved to hear that we had got the interview that they agreed to pay.

The plan had always been to drive from Las Vegas to California in a Tesla, both to experience the product which Elon Musk said would change the way we travel and to get some vital footage for our piece. So in the evening we collected a car from a showroom on the edge of town and set off on the 270-mile road trip to Los Angeles.

Even for someone with very little interest in cars, sitting behind the wheel of a top-of-the-range Model S P100D was an exhilarating experience. The acceleration was startling – even though we decided not to activate so-called Ludicrous mode, which would apparently have taken us from 0 to 60mph in under 3 seconds, outpacing a Ferrari or a Lamborghini. We were even more impressed by the rectangular touchscreen control pad, which made the car feel like a giant smartphone – indeed, part of the appeal was that you could install regular software updates which would improve certain features of the car.

But most of all we wanted to try out its autonomous driving capabilities. Elon Musk had made it clear that not only did he want to turn the car industry on its head by bringing an affordable yet attractive electric vehicle to the masses – something the forthcoming Model 3 would achieve – but he also planned to make his cars fully self-driving.

A couple of weeks earlier Musk had told *Fortune* magazine that this would not be too hard: 'I think we have all the pieces, and it's just about refining those pieces, putting them in place, and making sure they work across a huge number of environments – and then we're done. It's a much easier problem than people think it is.' He conceded that such a project would need thousands of people, but reckoned it could take a couple of years. Already autonomous features were being built into Teslas with a system called Autopilot, which you activated by pressing down on the control stalk. Autopilot would then take over the steering, keeping the car in lane and braking if it got too close to the vehicle in front. You could also pull out to overtake – just signal, and it would check that it was safe to change lanes.

In the race to build a self-driving car Tesla faced a formidable opponent in Google, which had been pouring vast sums into its autonomous vehicle project, soon to be renamed Waymo, since 2009. While in 2014 Google had unveiled the Firefly, a cute little autonomous car without a steering wheel, its approach centred on installing hardware and software into existing vehicles such as Chrysler Pacifica minivans.

Both firms depended on collecting vast amounts of data to refine their autonomous systems, and while Google used a lot of simulations as well as on-the-road testing, Tesla had the advantage of an army of testers in the form of its customers. Every journey they made, with or without Autopilot engaged, helped to provide more information about how the car might handle all sorts of road conditions. Every car was, in effect, a giant smartphone with a data connection with Tesla HQ so that it could receive software updates and send data back about its operations.

As we headed down the freeway in the dark, my producer Jat Gill added to that data. He briefly engaged Autopilot and the car started steering itself, staying within the white lines. But as we headed higher into the hills that straddle the border between Nevada and California, the conditions worsened and snow began to fall – quite a shock after a few days in balmy Las Vegas. After a nervy moment when the car suddenly decided it needed to follow some white lines heading off the freeway at an exit, Jat wrenched back the wheel from the robot and took firm control until we reached our destination for the night, a motel just over the border in California.

The following day, we drove to have breakfast at a nearby recharging station and emerged after 45 minutes to find that nothing had happened: we still had only 20 miles of battery life left. A call to Tesla revealed that this was a software issue. They sent a patch to the car via the cellular network, and soon we were charging properly, while reflecting again on the positives and negatives of a car that was essentially a smartphone on wheels.

The next task was to fill the car with GoPro cameras and set about getting some footage on our way to meet Elon Musk. This time, I was at the wheel of the Tesla, while the producer and the cameraman were in another car filming me. I activated the Autopilot for a while, and even tried out the overtaking feature, but I rested my trembling hands on the steering wheel and the whole experience felt less relaxing than being in full control. The technology seemed magical, and perhaps the robot software was a better driver than me but, I reflected, winning the trust of millions of motorists – along with the cyclists, pedestrians and others who would need to share the roads with autonomous vehicles – might prove quite a challenge.

A few hours later we were drawing into the car park at the Tesla Design centre in Hawthorne, on the fringes of Los Angeles Airport and just around the corner from the headquarters of SpaceX, Elon Musk's other extraordinarily exciting company.

Inside, we found a space that more than matched our expectations – the designer lair of either a creative genius or a Bond villain. To one side, purposeful engineers and software designers gathered in front of rows of giant iMacs, chewing over some meaty problem. To the other, several prototype vehicles were covered in dust sheets, hidden from our prying eyes. Just one, a Model S P100D like the one we had been driving, was uncovered as a prop for the background of our interview. In another corner we caught a glimpse of James Bond's Lotus Esprit from *The Spy Who Loved Me*, bought by Musk a couple of years earlier. No pictures, we were told – like most of what we saw, it was off limits to our cameras.

We had 90 minutes to prepare, ample time for cameraman Steve Adrain to set up lights and make everything look perfect. We tried to engage some of the engineers in conversation about the company, and found them amiable but evasive. So the tension mounted as I reflected that this interview had been three months in the planning and I needed to deliver the goods.

Suddenly, Musk was there, a surprisingly quiet and unassuming presence, quite different from what I had expected. The interview began, and for the first three or four minutes my anxiety rose. He spoke quietly, in something of a monotone and without animation. Nothing leaped out as a possible soundbite for a news piece.

Then, as we talked about his mission to transform the car industry, things began to liven up. 'The two biggest revolutions in transport are electrification and autonomy,' said Musk. 'Those are the two biggest innovations since the moving production line, and they're both happening about the same time.' When I asked him to look forward ten years, he predicted that full autonomy would have arrived, and choosing to drive would be a somewhat eccentric choice, something for which he had a striking phrase: 'Owning a car that is not self-driving in the long term will be like owning a horse – you would own it and use it for sentimental reasons, but not for daily use.'

Our conversation went on to roam far and wide. Apple was definitely going to make a car – it was 'an open secret'. (It has not happened yet.) Tesla needed to make a car that most people could afford if it was to make a substantial impact on the world. (If you think the Model 3 at £42,000 is affordable, then he has achieved that.) While we should not be concerned about the AI in Teslas – 'the car's not going to develop consciousness' – we needed to worry a lot about artificial intelligence leading to machines developing a will of their own: a scenario which was going to come 'faster than anyone appreciates'.

Near the end, in response to a question about what drove him, Musk came up with this: 'There are some things that are important for the future: sustainable energy, obviously; sustainable transport; ultimately becoming a multi-planet species and travelling out there among the stars.'

A multi-planet species? *Travelling among the stars?* Job done, I thought. But in some ways the best was yet to come. We had over-run our allotted time, but Musk graciously agreed to stay another five minutes while we got some shots to complete our package – the roughly two-and-a-half-minute report we would offer to the TV bulletins, with a much longer cut of the interview available online.

Musk and I stood chatting around the Model S, with the tycoon pointing out various features of the car. Then he told me about a new feature released in the last 24 hours: a smartphone app called Summon. This would allow Tesla owners to call their cars to them: 'The car will exit the garage, close the garage behind it, and come over to you.'

Wow, that sounded impressive.

But, said Musk, this was just the first 'baby step' of Summon. 'Ultimately you'll be able to summon the car from New York if you're living in LA, and it will drive across the country, charge itself at the various locations and come to you.'

But that must surely be a long way off? I stuttered.

The Tesla founder shrugged his shoulders. 'Not that long,' he said. 'A couple of years.'

That sounded hugely ambitious, I thought to myself – just imagine the technological advances and regulatory changes that would be needed to allow a car to drive on its own for 3,000 miles, only stopping to plug itself into a Tesla Supercharger . . .

But what a great line! What a brilliant example of the vaulting ambition of a man who refused to believe there were limits to what he and his company might achieve. I had one concern – had we actually recorded the conversation about Summon? After all, this was not part of the formal interview. Steve Adrain had been wandering around getting cutaway shots of the car, rather than focusing on what we were saying.

We packed up our equipment and hurried back to our Los Angeles hotel to check through what we had filmed. To my great relief, Elon Musk's outlandish prediction was there loud and clear, and even though the camera was either on a long shot or pointing at something else while he was talking, we could make it work. We emailed London to tell our bosses we had some great material and flew home overnight the next day, arriving both exhausted and exhilarated, planning to edit our various pieces and roll them out on the Monday evening.

On Monday morning my radio came on at 0630 with a huge story. David Bowie had died. Now, it is the guilty secret of every journalist that their first reaction on hearing of some major news event is not like that of any normal well-adjusted person. If they are not occupied with something else, they will ask how they can climb aboard this story. But if they've got a major piece of work, months in the planning, that is due to land that day, then, oblivious of the bigger picture, they will just curse their own bad luck.

It was clear to me that no editor in the BBC newsroom was going to be interested in anything that day but David Bowie. Yes, we could push our Elon Musk material out online but, despite the growing consensus that digital outlets were now more important than tired old analogue TV, we knew that deep down our bosses still believed that anything that did not appear on the *Six O'Clock* or *Ten O'Clock News* had not really happened.

But while the bulletins through the day were wall-to-wall Bowie, at one meeting in the afternoon a very senior person spoke up in favour of a bit of variety oblivious of the bigger picture – or so we heard later. The Director of News, James Harding, who had long been a fan of more technology coverage and made frequent trips to Silicon Valley, made it clear that space should be found in the *Ten O'Clock News* running order for Elon Musk.

We were the final item, but also made it as a headline. That meant we could run all of our online material, including an extended cut of the interview, a news story and a blog about the experience of meeting the Tesla tycoon. In the blogpost, I focused on that outlandish prediction about a car driving itself across the United States within a couple of years. I wrote that it was 'bonkers' to think that this could be achieved so quickly, but went on, 'Elon Musk is both bonkers and brilliant, the most visionary technology leader I have encountered in 20 years of interviewing many of the leading figures in the industry.'

'Bonkers but Brilliant' was also the headline of the piece, and it is safe to say it did not go down well with its subject. Within hours an email was winging its way across the Atlantic from Elon Musk's smart and amiable young PR chief, with whom we had had a good relationship until then. The headline, he said, was 'frankly just disrespectful', and did not reflect the spirit of what was otherwise a great interview. I wrote back to suggest that there had been a misunderstanding: on this side of the Atlantic 'bonkers' could be affectionate, and could mean something that was crazy but at the same time possible – for example, 'That idea is bonkers but it might just work.'

I am not sure my explanation worked – certainly, I have never since been able to arrange another interview with Elon Musk. I also got my first flavour of his growing army of social media fans. Plenty of his devoted followers left comments on the YouTube video I had put up of the uncut interview, suggesting I was just too dumb to understand the great man's vision, and had not deserved to meet him. But the truth was that in January 2016, nine years after seeing Steve Jobs unveil the iPhone, I was convinced that I had met someone who could bring the world another leap forward, and with technology that might have a much greater impact on the way we lived.

The next few years were, however, to prove turbulent for Elon Musk, and would also sap some of the optimism about the progress that could be made towards his vision of sustainable transport and energy, let alone the journey towards being a multi-planet species.

As far as building an affordable electric car went, and turning Tesla into a company that could challenge the traditional powerhouses of the automobile industry in Detroit, Tokyo and Munich, the scorecard was largely positive. The Model 3 – undoubtedly one of those cars lurking under the black sheets when we did our interview – was unveiled later in 2016 to huge excitement. Within a week more than 300,000 people had reserved one. That meant potential sales of $14 billion if all those who had put down a $1,000 deposit followed through and bought the car. That promised to transform the economics of a company that throughout its life had been like one of its cars after a 200-mile trip: close to running out of juice. Its losses in 2016 were $675 million; the following year they would triple to nearly $2 billion as the firm poured cash into the mass production of the Model 3. It was Tesla's good fortune to have been pursuing its mission to transform motoring at a time when shareholders and the venture capital industry – in the United States at least – were extraordinarily patient with technology companies which racked up huge losses. With interest rates at record lows, companies like Uber or Peter Thiel's data firm Palantir were allowed to postpone profitability for years by investors counting on huge returns if their dreams of market dominance came off.

And in the summer of 2017 there was good news from Tesla. The first Model 3s were delivered to buyers and, despite some initial production hiccups, by the summer of 2019 the vehicle had captured 67 per cent of sales of electric cars in the United States and was beginning to conquer other markets around the world. What had not happened, either at Tesla or at other companies, was the rapid progress towards fully autonomous driving that had seemed possible – and indeed had been promised in the marketing material for the affordable car.

The Model 3 may have been cheaper than previous Teslas, but it came with the same Autopilot technology. 'Eight surround cameras provide 360 degrees of visibility around the car at up to 250 meters of range,' explained the Tesla website.

Twelve updated ultrasonic sensors complement this vision, allowing for detection of both hard and soft objects at nearly twice the distance of the prior system. A forward-facing radar with enhanced processing provides additional data about the world on a redundant wavelength that is able to see through heavy rain, fog, dust and even the car ahead.

The online manual went on to promise 'full self-driving capabilities in the future – through software updates designed to improve functionality over time.' And in October 2019 Musk told investors that full self-driving could be available within months, to Tesla owners who had paid for an upgrade package costing $7,000.

But by this time, Autopilot had a big PR problem. The whole point of the move to autonomous driving was that it would make cars much safer, and lives would be saved. But soon there was evidence that on the path to full autonomy driving could become more dangerous.

The industry had developed a five-stage route map to chart the process by which humans would gradually be eliminated from driving. Level 1 meant some limited driver assistance through features such as adaptive cruise control; level 2 meant more automation, though the motorist had to have their eyes on the road at all times. Level 3 would see the car capable of driving itself in good weather conditions, but in limited environments such as in dedicated lanes on motorways, with the driver free to take their hands off the wheel and their eyes off the road, but ready to take over if needed. At level 4 the driver only really needed to enter the destination, and the car would drive itself, although it might decide that it did not want to go out in the snow, or that the backstreets of Paris or London were too tricky. And level 5 would be full automation: a vehicle that might not even have a steering wheel, allowing you to watch a movie or fall asleep in the back.

Now, Autopilot was probably at level 2, but some Tesla owners seemed to think that it was at 4 or even 5. A few videos showed drivers snoozing at the wheel, or even sitting in the passenger seat. And then in May 2016 there was the first fatality.

Joshua Brown, a tech entrepreneur and Tesla enthusiast, had posted several videos on YouTube showing his car in Autopilot mode. One, which was promoted on Twitter by Elon Musk, shows the feature helping to avoid a collision with a truck. But just three weeks afterwards, Brown died after his Tesla collided with a truck and trailer that was crossing a Florida freeway. It seemed that the car's sensors had failed to spot the white truck against the bright sky.

Tesla put out a blogpost in which it sought to blame everything but its own technology for the tragic accident. It was the first fatality in over 130 million miles driven with Autopilot activated. The system came with clear instructions on its safe use, gave drivers frequent alerts if they took their hands off the wheel, and slowed the car to a halt if they ignored the warnings.

Other accidents followed, and Tesla faced mounting criticism over the labelling of its driver-assistance feature. Thatcham Research, which works for the British insurance industry, brought out a report claiming that labels like Autopilot could confuse drivers into believing their cars were more capable than was in fact the case. 'There's a problem with the manufacturers trying to introduce technology and consumers not being ready for it, not being sure if it's automated or "Do I need to keep watching?"' said Thatcham's Matthew Avery. 'We want it very clear. Either you are driving – assisted – or you're not driving – automated.' He took me out onto a test track in Oxfordshire to prove the point. He drove a Tesla in Autopilot mode behind another car which halted when it encountered standing traffic – and our car pulled up safely too. We went round again, but this time the car we were following pulled out at the last moment when it encountered the traffic jam – and our Tesla carried on, crashing into a dummy car, which disintegrated.

Tesla was not the only firm to suffer an autonomous driving accident. Phoenix, Arizona, with its quiet streets laid out in a grid and its balmy weather, had become the testing ground for a number of the firms wanting to trial self-driving cars. Among them was Uber, the taxi-hailing app which was pouring huge sums into its research programme, buying up small AI start-ups and hiring most of the robotics department from Carnegie Mellon University. Its rapid expansion around the globe had seen it rack up huge losses, and some analysts thought its only route to profit lay in taking away the drivers.

Late one evening in March 2018, a woman was pushing a bicycle across a dual carriageway in a Phoenix suburb when she was struck and killed by an Uber test vehicle in autonomous mode. There was a safety driver behind the wheel, but it soon emerged that she was watching a TV show on her phone in the moments before the crash.

The report into the accident by the National Safety Transportation Board (NTSB) was also damning about the autonomous driving software. It said the Uber car was travelling at 43 miles per hour when it first detected the woman six seconds before the impact. 'As the vehicle and pedestrian paths converged, the self-driving system software classified the pedestrian as an unknown object, as a vehicle, and then as a bicycle, with varying expectations of future travel path. At 1.3 seconds before impact, the self-driving system determined that an emergency braking manoeuvre was needed to mitigate a collision.' An emergency braking system had been turned off, with Uber insisting that it relied on the human operator to intervene in circumstances like this. The final report from the NTSB zeroed in on what it called 'automation complacency': the problem of humans having excessive confidence in the robot driving system, just as Thatcham Research had said.

Two things were becoming clear. Even if the AI behind self-driving cars was 95 per cent there, the final 5 per cent was going to be very challenging. Teaching a robot driver to recognize a pedestrian pushing a bicycle or a white truck silhouetted against a bright sky might prove more time-consuming than asking it to become a world champion Go player.

And the other problem was what you might call the messy middle of that five-stage route to full automation. Asking a human to be alert and ready to take over the wheel in a Level 3 car, which was perfectly capable of driving itself most of the time, was already proving to be dangerous.

In 2019 I visited the Phoenix area to make a radio documentary about the progress towards autonomous driving. Remember, by then – if what Elon Musk had told me in 2016 was right – Teslas should have been making their way solo across the United States. And even if that had been a bit optimistic, others thought the autonomous future was within our grasp. In his 2017 Budget the UK Chancellor of the Exchequer, Philip Hammond, had promised that driverless cars would be on British roads by 2021. When I emailed a Treasury official to ask whether that really meant an autonomous vehicle with no safety driver the answer came back in block capitals: YES – THIS WOULD MEAN FULL SELF-DRIVING CARS WITH NOBODY BEHIND THE WHEEL. In retrospect, this seems optimistic, to say the least.

In Arizona I did find one example of a fully autonomous vehicle. A robotics company called Nuro was delivering groceries from a Scottsdale store in a tiny truck with two compartments which you unlocked with a smartphone app when it trundled up your drive with the shopping. (This trial project was discontinued the following year.) But my main focus was the world's first robot taxi service, which had just been launched by Google's Waymo. While Uber had been forced to abandon its autonomous driving trial in Arizona after the crash, Waymo was forging ahead. Its test vehicles had already driven 10 million miles on public roads, and now it was confident enough to start charging for rides.

We first took a trip with a Waymo PR executive – and a safety driver – around some quiet back streets. The technology was impressive, with a screen showing us what the software was seeing: cyclists, pedestrians on the sidewalk, other cars approaching. After a while, as we slowly made our way at under 20mph back to the Waymo depot, it even became a little boring, so capable was the technology.

Then we took a ride with a customer, however, and things got interesting. Shaun Metz was one of a few hundred locals selected to test Waymo One, the robot taxi service. It worked just like Uber: you chose your destination in the app, and a car arrived and took you there all on its own. Well, not quite. There was still a safety driver behind the wheel. Ryan told us he and his wife used the service for weekly visits to the grocery store, in places with limited parking, or for nights out: 'We're hoping to go from a two-vehicle to a one-vehicle household eventually, and optimistic this technology might get us there.'

But as we headed along the freeway on the 20-minute ride to his office things began to go wrong. As we approached our exit there was a solid line of traffic to our right. An assertive human driver would probably have squeezed over into the next lane and made it to the exit ramp – but the robot, which cannot exceed the speed limit, was more cautious. The car missed that exit and the next one before finally leaving the freeway. And when we were back on the suburban streets it appeared to freeze at a junction where it needed to turn left across traffic – after a while the engineer behind the wheel had to take over and complete the turn. Waymo's software appeared to have been programmed to be ultra-cautious – understandable in the context of the Uber accident. I came away from that trip sceptical about just how soon the streets of a city like London would be filled with self-driving cars.

Elon Musk, meanwhile, was still thinking big, with both SpaceX and Tesla the canvases on which he painted exciting visions of the future. SpaceX continued to astound and delight with its live-streamed launches and mostly successful rocket landings, and Musk had a new idea called Starlink. This would involve launching up to 42,000 mini satellites into orbit – eclipsing the 5,000 satellites already up there – to offer superfast broadband to far-flung places. He had suggested this could be extremely profitable, providing funds for even more ambitious projects such as a city on Mars. Sceptics warned that the Earth could be encircled by a layer of space junk, while astronomers claimed the satellites would outnumber visible stars, harming scientific observation. By October 2020, Starlink had over 700 satellites in orbit and Musk was talking of launching a trial internet service in the northern United States and Canada. Profits were naturally a distant prospect, although he speculated that the small investors who had poured their money into Tesla might be eager to get a stake in this venture if he floated it.

Another of his obsessions involved urban transport. Frustrated by the traffic jams in Los Angeles, he launched a subsidiary of SpaceX called the Boring Company, promising to build tunnels to speed traffic beneath and between cities. He insisted that he could revolutionize tunnelling technology just as he was transforming the motor industry. One idea was to build on a concept called the Hyperloop, a kind of vacuum tube along which shuttles would be projected at up to 700mph. Musk had originally said he was too busy with other things and urged others to adopt his idea, so Richard Branson's Virgin Hyperloop One built a 500-metre test track in Nevada, which I visited in 2017. There was heady talk of hyperloops between London's Gatwick and Heathrow Airports, or even replacing the UK's long-delayed HS2 high-speed rail project with a hyperloop system – but the years passed without much evidence of Virgin signing commercial deals.

In the meantime, Elon Musk was announcing all sorts of ambitious hyperloop plans: a tunnel crossing Los Angeles in five minutes when a car above ground would take 45 minutes; another connecting New York and Washington DC. There was a 1-mile test tunnel in LA and a glossy video showing a car – a Tesla, naturally – being lowered underground in an elevator, loaded onto a sort of skateboard and then shot through the tube to its destination. Cynics, especially those from cities with decent underground public transport systems, wondered whether this was anything more than a billionaire's fantasy. But the Boring Company did sign a contract with the city of Las Vegas, albeit for a relatively modest project to build a tunnel under the Convention Centre.

All through this period from 2016 to 2020, Musk's main focus was on Tesla. It was an extraordinarily turbulent time, with the company lurching from triumph to disaster and back again: at one stage looking like it was about to run out of money, at another seeing its share price soar to a level which made it overtake Toyota as the world's most valuable car company. This appeared ludicrous. Tesla was able to announce its first annual profit when it reported results in July 2020, selling 368,000 cars and earning revenues of $24.6 billion. But over the same period, Toyota sold nearly 9 million cars and earned $279 billion in revenue and, like Tesla, managed to stay profitable during the pandemic. Its share price driven sky-high by excitable small investors, Tesla's valuation implied that it would soon overtake a business currently earning ten times as much revenue. However unlikely that seemed, it showed that plenty of people did buy into Elon Musk's optimistic view of our technology future, even at a time of general gloom about the state of the world.

Here was a man confronting the big challenges of our time. His beautiful and ever more innovative electric cars were forcing the whole automobile industry to contemplate the end of the internal combustion engine and, along with his advances in battery technology, promised to make a significant contribution to the fight against climate change. His dreams of interplanetary travel and a settlement on Mars may have seemed far-fetched, but in May 2020 the SpaceX *Dragon Endeavour* took NASA astronauts to the International Space Station on the first commercial-crewed mission. From now on, Musk looked set to play a leading role in America's renewed programme of space exploration.

And yet, here is the irony. This man who promised to give us what Peter Thiel had dreamed of – yes, Musk did unveil a plan for a flying car, promising to integrate SpaceX technology into his Tesla Roadster – was nearly brought to earth by 140 characters. At key moments his obsession with Twitter plunged his company into crisis and inflicted severe damage on his reputation.

In the summer of 2018, with the world transfixed by the fate of a group of Thai schoolboys trapped in a cave, the Tesla founder waded in, offering a mini submarine to help with the rescue. This did not impress a British diver, Vernon Unsworth, who was helping with the rescue, and a war of words broke out when he suggested Musk should 'stick his submarine where it hurts'. Without any evidence, the Tesla tycoon then suggested Mr Unsworth was a child abuser, calling him 'pedo guy' on Twitter.

Musk had used his social media platform, where he had 22 million followers, to attack an obscure individual who was involved in a desperate mission to save lives. Even though he later successfully defended himself against a defamation suit, the incident seemed to many to show an unpleasant arrogance and lack of judgement in a man with lofty ambitions to advance humanity.

But if anyone thought he had learned a lesson about the dangers of social media, they were soon to be disappointed. One day in August 2018 Musk tweeted this: 'Am considering taking Tesla private at $420. Funding secured.' He was telling the world, and in particular his shareholders, that he was going to buy out the company, whose shares were then trading at around $340, at a premium. What is more, he had the money lined up. The tweet came as Musk was knee-deep in what he himself described as the 'hell' of ramping up Model 3 production, a process on which the survival of the company depended. Moreover, making an announcement about a public company which could move the market is governed by extremely strict rules, and tweeting it out is not in the rulebook. Even worse, it turned out that it was not true that he had the money lined up, even if he had been in talks with Saudi Arabia's sovereign wealth fund. The Securities and Exchange Commission was not amused. The watchdog sued him, and eventually Musk had to step down as chairman of Tesla and agree to have any future tweets reviewed by the company's lawyers.

For a while that appeared to tame him. Yet as the coronavirus pandemic took hold, it seemed to unleash his worst instincts once more. Whether it was raging against the lockdown which shut his Fremont factory, and predicting in March that by the end of April there would be 'close to zero' new coronavirus cases in the United States, or declaring that Tesla's share price was too high, or that his girlfriend, the musician Grimes, was mad at him, he continued to tweet an often obnoxious picture of himself. In Elon Musk, then, we have the personification of this smartphone social era. A man who embodies the triumph of technology, with a grand vision of a world transformed – where the computer in your pocket would summon your car to you from across the continent, or maybe book you a ticket on the next flight to Mars.

And he was also the guy who would get into a rage on Twitter and pick a fight which nearly destroyed everything he had spent a decade building.

The research firm Gartner has what it calls a Hype Cycle to describe the progress of any new technology. At first it soars to the peak of inflated expectations, then plunges down into the trough of disillusionment, only finally climbing the slope of enlightenment to end up on the plateau of productivity. In the next section of this book we are heading downhill for a while, trying not to get too depressed about what these wonderful new tools have done to our brains, our relationships and our society.

Part II

Things Fall Apart

7

The Woes of the Web

It was a rainy night in East London in July 2012. But for 80,000 people packed into a new stadium the mood was exuberant, and around the world hundreds of millions of people were caught up in the excitement. A very modern but also very British pageant was under way, masterminded by a movie director with a gift for telling stories that were both accessible and profound.

The opening ceremony for the London Olympics, directed by Danny Boyle, featured a series of *tableaux vivants* with a huge cast. Giant chimneys sprang from the turf in the middle of the stadium to illustrate the Industrial Revolution; nurses danced on hospital beds to celebrate Britain's National Health Service. We even saw the Queen, escorted by James Bond, parachute from a helicopter into the stadium to appear moments later in the Royal Box. Or so it seemed.

Then suddenly the spotlight was on a balding, middle-aged man sitting at a computer tapping out a message, which flashed around the stadium on a strip of LED lights attached to every seat. It read, 'This is for everyone,' and was actually a tweet which went out to the world.

American television commentators were bemused. 'If you haven't heard of him', said NBC's Meredith Viera, 'we haven't either.' Her colleague Matt Lauer instructed viewers to 'google him.'

If they had done so, they would have discovered that it was the man at the computer who had made it possible for them to google; indeed, it was he who had ushered in the digital era.

Back in 1989, Tim Berners-Lee was working at the CERN particle physics lab near Geneva, when he drafted a memo about an idea to improve collaboration between scientists at CERN and their counterparts around the world. 'Vague but exciting', his boss scrawled on the document, and two years later that idea, the World Wide Web, was born. It turned the internet from a niche and nerdy backwater into a global communication system, the vital infrastructure on which our way of life now depends.

The message that Berners-Lee tapped out on the evening of the opening ceremony on a NeXt computer he had used at CERN referred not just to the Olympics but to the technology he had invented. By 2012, 1 billion people around the world had a smartphone, and a few months after the Olympics, Facebook announced that it now had more than a billion daily active users. The social smartphone era had truly arrived.

Sir Tim – he had been knighted in 2004 – had always been a utopian when it came to the power of the Web to give people the freedom to express themselves. From the start he had seen it as a 'read/write platform': in other words, a medium in which everyone could create content, rather than a broadcast model, where there were millions of passive users just sitting back and absorbing what a few giant corporations decided was interesting.

At first that had failed to materialize – for most people the Web was still about reading rather than writing. But putting powerful computers in people's pockets with all sorts of creativity tools, and giving them social media platforms where they could express themselves, changed that, and began to make Berners-Lee's vision seem more credible.

The Olympics was a good example of how things had changed. What had once been an event most of us only experienced through the lens of what the broadcasters chose to show us now became a huge social media happening. Tim Berners-Lee's 'This is for everyone' tweet kicked things off, and there followed an explosion of photos and memes, commentary and jokes, from athletes and celebrities, but also from anyone who felt like celebrating the event. One example – a photo of a Venezuelan fencing gold medallist travelling back to the Olympic Village on the Docklands Light Railway – went viral, capturing the democratic spirit of the games.

Looking back, it feels as though this was the high point of our optimism about what the Web, smartphones and social media could do for us. Ever since, we have woken up to the power of the giant corporations behind smartphones and the Web, we have asked what these tools are doing to our democracy, to our children, to our brains – and we have liked the answers less and less. Hope about what this personal technology revolution could do for us has been replaced by fear. And you can see that descent into gloom personified in the way the views of the Web's creator about his brainchild have changed.

Over the last 20 years, I must have interviewed Tim Berners-Lee about a dozen times. It is always a privilege – after all, he is probably the most influential Briton of the last 50 years. When I first met him, I told him that my oldest son, then still in primary school, knew all about him because he had read a children's book all about this wonderful inventor called Tim. Once, I took along as a producer a woman who had started her career in the BBC as an engineer and was completely starstruck. Berners-Lee graciously agreed to a photo with her, and she later told me it was one of the most exciting days of her life.

But interviewing Sir Tim in the hope of getting a soundbite was a fool's errand. Words, phrases, random thoughts seemed to tumble out of him in a staccato torrent. It was almost as if he was the living embodiment of the World Wide Web, hopping from one link to another at breakneck speed.

For many years, however, there was a constant theme in our conversations. The Web was a force for good, attempts to regulate it were largely futile, and the more freely information flowed across it, the more data we shared, the better. 'I imagined the Web as an open platform that would allow everyone, everywhere to share information, access opportunities and collaborate across geographic and cultural boundaries,' Sir Tim wrote in 2017. And in an interview for this book he remembered that for a long time he and his collaborators had been focused on just a few things: 'Freedom, connectivity, bandwidth – just more, more, more metaweb. More web was better.'

In March 2019 I met Sir Tim at CERN in Switzerland for an interview to mark the thirtieth anniversary of that first 'vague but exciting' memo outlining his idea for the Web. He was at the start of a 40-hour journey that would see him travel to London's Science Museum and then on to Lagos in Nigeria for events marking this momentous anniversary. He seemed to be in a playful mood – we filmed some set-up shots with him in the CERN data centre which was the backdrop for the interview and, when I got my phone out to take some video, he produced his and started filming me filming him. He told me how he'd plugged the very first Web server into the centre's uninterruptible power supply over Christmas in 1990 so that nobody would switch it off – only for the whole place to be powered down.

But this time much of the interview was anything but celebratory. He talked of the Web's downward plunge towards a dysfunctional future, of 'large swathes of people being very nasty to each other' on social media, of concerns about privacy and about the manipulation of the democratic process. When I ended with a question about whether the overall impact of the web had been good, I expected an upbeat answer. Instead, gesturing to indicate an upward and then a downward curve, he said that after a good first 15 years, things had turned bad, and a 'mid-course correction' was needed.

In this and in a couple of other interviews I had with Sir Tim in the next year, two words kept coming up when I asked him what the signal had been that things were going wrong. Those words were 'Cambridge' and 'Analytica'.

I first heard of that company in November 2016, just a day after Donald Trump defeated Hillary Clinton in the contest to become the 45th President of the United States. A press release headlined 'Digital Campaigning Reaches New Heights in 2016 Election' arrived in my inbox.

It boasted that 'Cambridge Analytica's Digital Team' had 'planned and executed the digital advertising strategy that won over undecided voters for President-elect Trump.' The firm had carried out thousands of highly targeted advertising campaigns across Facebook, Twitter and other platforms. Cambridge Analytica had 'pioneered an innovative collaboration of data-driven targeting methods to ensure that all key voters were reached with the campaign's messages', hunting down the undecided and then dividing them into 12–15 subgroups to receive highly targeted messages. 'Our cutting-edge digital capabilities allowed the campaign to reach voters more effectively than ever before, and at a fraction of the cost spent by the Democratic candidate,' said the firm's chief executive Alexander Nix.

This sounded like a great story. I had been interested in the technology of election campaigning for a while. During the UK's 2010 General Election I had been given the title of Digital Election Correspondent, and asked to monitor the campaigns and find out how they were using the latest modern methods. While the parties all talked of learning from Barack Obama's 2008 campaign, thought to have broken new ground in communicating online with millions of voters, there was little evidence of that. Yes, the Conservatives bought up a few Google search terms, the Liberal Democrats had a popular Facebook page, and there was a frenzy of tweeting during the TV debates from politicos who had just discovered this new medium. But apart from heavier use of email databases, it had turned out to be quite an old-fashioned campaign, dominated by TV debates, the unveiling of posters and daily press conferences.

By 2015, when the Conservatives spent £1.2 million on Facebook ads during their successful General Election campaign, compared to Labour's paltry £16,500, things had moved on a bit. It is interesting to note that few politicians seemed concerned at that time at the power that tech giants such as Facebook and Google were beginning to wield over elections – just keen to learn how they could use it to benefit them.

The Conservative MP Damian Collins, who was later to be one of the social network's fiercest inquisitors, remembers noticing the change in its role in elections. 'Facebook was a niche thing that was seen as a supplement to traditional forms of campaigning. It very quickly flipped to being the main channel through which campaigns were won.'

Of course, American election spending is on a wholly different scale from what we see in the UK. In 2016 the Donald Trump campaign spent close to $90 million on Facebook ads. Up until the result the focus by the pundits had been not on paid advertising but on Facebook's potential to spread misinformation – what had rapidly become known as Fake News. But with that press release from Cambridge Analytica came the first realization that it might have been the micro-targeting of ads on the social media platform that had swung the election. So we wanted to hear more about this on my weekly World Service radio programme *Tech Tent*. We asked the company's PR person whether we could get hold of Alexander Nix or another senior executive. After a bit of to and fro, it appeared that they were too busy celebrating, so we ended up with what appeared to be the last person left in the headquarters of the Trump digital operation in San Antonio, Texas.

David Wilkinson was a young British data scientist who had spent six months on the campaign, and seemed very excited about what it had achieved. He told us where their vast data collection had come from.

> We had demographic and political data very kindly provided to us by the Republican Party itself. And we also have our own commercial data like consumer habits, purchase histories and things like that for every American voter. Then we have the campaign's data. So those are supporter lists, email lists, donors, and then finally we conducted our own research projects through the campaign.

Oh, but they did not just have this huge data pool. They had Cambridge Analytica's magic sauce . . . 'Machine learning and data science' had allowed them to tie all these data points together in a subtle way. 'So we knew who was the most persuadable, who needed encouragement to get out and vote.'

While it all sounded very clever, I tried to probe this young man to find out if he had any thoughts about the politics of using these techniques to elect a man like Trump. But he started talking about late-night pizza and camaraderie, as if it had all been just another hackathon.

We also featured in that week's programme Mark Zuckerberg's reaction when he was challenged about the role misinformation had played in the election. This comment at a conference came back to bite him: 'Personally I think the idea that fake news on Facebook, which is a very small amount of the content, influenced the election in any way – I think is a pretty crazy idea. Voters make decisions based on their lived experience.'

There was plenty of criticism, and a growing sense that Mark Zuckerberg was either naive or reckless about the impact of his empire on democracy. But at that stage, nobody was really connecting the dots between Facebook and the data manipulation employed by Cambridge Analytica. The row over the election receded, and throughout 2017 the social network's audience continued to grow and its share price scaled new heights. In June of that year, Facebook's monthly users topped 2 billion for the first time, with nearly three-quarters accessing it via a mobile phone. Whatever the privacy campaigners said, most people seemed comfortable – if they even thought about it – with a deal whereby they handed over a certain amount of data in exchange for a free service.

But in March 2018, a British newspaper blew a great big hole in all of those comfortable assumptions. 'Revealed: 50 million Facebook profiles harvested for Cambridge Analytica in major data breach', read the headline in the *Observer* on a story by Carole Cadwalladr. The journalist had been chipping away at the story of Cambridge Analytica for over a year, and had collaborated with the *New York Times*, which published its own story. She had hit paydirt when a former employee she had been talking to for months finally agreed to go on the record.

Christopher Wylie described how the firm had collaborated with a Cambridge University psychology researcher, Aleksandr Kogan, to scrape data from millions of Facebook users for use in its political campaign work. Dr Kogan had created a personality quiz app, thisisyourdigitallife, and invited Facebook users to take part. It collected valuable data, not just about those who had ticked a box to participate, but about millions of their Facebook friends too.

The data might sound reasonably innocuous, consisting mainly of Facebook users' locations and 'likes', the pages on the social network in which they had expressed an interest. But other Cambridge psychologists had demonstrated that from such data you could draw all sorts of conclusions about everything from sexual orientation to political persuasion. And when Cambridge Analytica merged this with the wealth of other data it had acquired from legitimate sources, it enabled the microtargeting of voters with individually crafted messages. People in Florida who had liked the National Rifle Association's page might get an advert warning the Democrats would take their guns, while their neighbours who liked a particular brand of car would be told that Republican policies would cut the price of gasoline.

Facebook's first reaction on hearing that this story was about to break was to threaten legal action against the *Observer* – a move even the company soon realized was dumb. Within days, America's Federal Trade Commission and the UK's Information Commissioner were launching investigations. Facebook's share price plunged 7 per cent in a day, wiping $36 billion off the company's value. Politicians on both sides of the Atlantic, some of whom had until recently been embarrassingly eager to hang out with Mark Zuckerberg, were now demanding he appear before Congressional and Parliamentary committees.

Three days after the *Observer* and the *New York Times* published their stories, and after a devastating undercover documentary by the UK's Channel 4 revealed how low Cambridge Analytica would stoop as it lent its services to election campaigns across the world, Zuckerberg felt obliged to pen a blogpost explaining what had happened.

Without ever quite saying sorry to the people whose data had been misused, he went through the history of the affair. In 2013, before Facebook tightened its rules on the data app developers could access, Aleksandr Kogan had created the app that had ended up collecting the data of tens of millions of users. In 2015 Facebook had been told by journalists at the *Guardian*, the *Observer*'s sister paper, that Kogan had shared data from his app with Cambridge Analytica. That was against the rules, so Kogan's app had been banned, and he and Cambridge Analytica had been told to delete all the data immediately.

So, wrote Zuckerberg, they had been shocked – *shocked* – to be told by the journalists a few days earlier that not all of that data had in fact been deleted. Now Facebook was going to launch a very serious investigation into which other apps might have been similarly reckless with user data. It would tighten restrictions further, and give users a tool to allow them to see which developers had access to their data. No word, though, on why Facebook had not told everyone about this illicit data-sharing the previous year – or why it had threatened the *Observer* with its lawyers just a few days ago.

It was not until the following month, when he was summoned to Washington for two days of Congressional hearings, that the Facebook founder made a full apology. 'It was my mistake, and I'm sorry,' he said. 'It's clear now that we didn't do enough to prevent these tools from being used for harm. That goes for fake news, foreign interference in elections, and hate speech, as well as developers and data privacy.'

Three thousand miles away, a British politician was watching the hearings with impatience. Damian Collins MP was chairman of the Digital, Culture and Media Select Committee of the House of Commons, which had launched an inquiry into fake news some months before, having decided that it was a growing problem. 'It wasn't just that there was disinformation on social media, but that the audience for that had grown to a level where it could be argued that it was crowding out real news and information.' The Facebook executives who had appeared in front of his committee seemed far too relaxed, he had found, about their role in spreading misinformation: 'Their view was that it wasn't their responsibility to identify the fact this activity was taking place,' he told me when we met in his House of Commons office in 2020. 'It wasn't their job to find this stuff, which seemed to be a big dereliction of responsibility on their part.'

Now, as Collins watched members of Congress each get just four minutes to question Facebook's founder, he was convinced his committee could provide a more forensic encounter. And as the scandal concerned the activities of a British company and a Cambridge University academic, surely it was right that Zuckerberg should make the trip to the Palace of Westminster to give evidence?

But, despite repeated requests, Damian Collins never got his way. The most senior executive Facebook would supply was its Chief Technology Officer, Mike Schroepfer, but his appearance in front of the committee, where he repeatedly said he would have to get back to them about various issues, did not satisfy the chairman. 'Later that same day we wrote back to him and Mark Zuckerberg with over forty questions where he [Schroepfer] wasn't able to answer.' Nevertheless, the committee persisted, taking evidence from Cambridge Analytica's Alexander Nix – he was recalled after it appeared he had been less than frank on his first appearance – from Aleksandr Kogan and from the whistleblower Christopher Wylie.

For Collins, and for many of those watching in the UK and around the world, it was Wylie's evidence that was the highlight. The BBC Parliamentary Correspondent Mark D'Arcy described it as 'by a distance, the most astounding thing I've seen in Parliament'. The young Canadian, his hair dyed pink, took the committee through the history of Cambridge Analytica's activities, making a string of remarkable allegations. He said the EU referendum had been won by fraud, accusing Vote Leave of channelling cash through AIQ, a Canadian firm linked to Cambridge Analytica. He described the dirty tricks used during a Nigerian election campaign, and even suggested that his predecessor at the company had died mysteriously in a Kenyan hotel room after a deal had gone sour. Some questioned

Wylie's motives – after all, it was he who had worked with Aleksandr Kogan to harvest data from Facebook. But Damian Collins says Wylie's evidence was devastating. 'He talked about what he knew, and then gave us documents that backed up what he said. People try to question Chris's motives for doing it – but I don't think anyone's ever come up with a serious rebuttal to the information that he put into the public domain.'

What had been an inquiry into the general issue of misinformation became increasingly focused on Facebook, with Damian Collins leading the charge. He repeatedly confronted and harried the company, not just over the issue of whether its chief executive would appear, but over its track record long before the Cambridge Analytica affair. At one stage he even used parliamentary powers few knew existed to seize a cache of Facebook internal documents he thought would throw a light on its murky past. The documents were in the possession of the boss of a small software firm, Six4Three, which was involved in a legal battle with Facebook. When this man travelled to London, Collins sent a Commons official, the Serjeant-at-Arms, to his hotel to demand he hand over the documents. When the businessman refused to do so, he was escorted to Parliament and told he risked prison if he did not comply with the order. He complied. 'We are in uncharted territory,' Collins told the *Guardian*. 'This is an unprecedented move, but it's an unprecedented situation. We've failed to get answers from Facebook, and we believe the documents contain information of very high public interest.'

There were rumblings by this time, particularly among Brexiteers whose conduct during the EU referendum had come under the committee's spotlight, that Damian Collins was out of control, or that he was unduly influenced by the *Observer* journalist Carole Cadwalladr. But he insists that beyond the political manoeuvring and the parliamentary shenanigans there was an issue of great concern to real people.

When you started to get into the fact that Facebook gathered data about what you did when you weren't on Facebook, and gathered data about non-Facebook customers, captured data from Android phones, people's text messages and calls, and that that data wasn't safe, could end up in the hands of people you'd never wanted to have that data, I think that's when people started to think, there's a problem here.

Eventually, the Select Committee produced two hefty, headline-making reports on its inquiry. Their interim report said the time had come for the tech giants to face greater scrutiny and regulation over the harmful content they put on their platforms. It made clear that their whole business model incentivized dodgy behaviour. 'Tech companies are not passive platforms on which users input content – they reward what is most engaging, because engagement is part of their business model and their growth strategy.' But rather than the relatively arcane debate about making the tech companies legally liable for the harmful content they published, it was the chairman's quotes about the threat to democracy that provided the lead story for broadcasters and the newspapers. In the press release accompanying the report Collins said, 'We are facing nothing less than a crisis in our democracy – based on the systematic manipulation of data to support the relentless targeting of citizens, without their consent, by campaigns of disinformation and messages of hate.'

A year later, the final report zeroed in on Facebook. In scathing terms, it denounced the company as 'digital gangsters', accusing its leaders of deliberately breaking privacy and competition laws, and obstructing the committee in its attempts to uncover the truth. Those documents seized from Six4Three were released alongside the report, with the committee claiming they reinforced its case that Facebook had been more concerned with marketing its users' data than protecting it. Among the revelations was the claim that Mark Zuckerberg and his colleagues exploited the data of Facebook users as a way of rewarding partner companies, while cutting out access to that information for rivals. So, for instance, Amazon, which was spending money on Facebook adverts, got access to data, while MessageMe, a fast-growing messaging app seen as competition, did not. In another case, when Twitter's short-lived Vine video platform was trying to use Facebook to let users find friends via the network, an executive sent the boss an email suggesting that it be shut out. 'Yup, go for it,' replied Zuckerberg.

This time Damian Collins issued a damning verdict on Facebook's founder. 'Mark Zuckerberg continually fails to show the levels of leadership and personal responsibility that should be expected from someone who sits at the top of one of the world's biggest companies.' The report also said that there was an urgent need to reform Britain's electoral laws so they were fit for the digital age, called for statutory regulation of Facebook and other tech giants, and demanded an independent investigation into foreign intervention and voter manipulation in the 2014 Scottish referendum.

So the Cambridge Analytica affair had been a turning point. It had resulted in the humbling of the most powerful company of the smartphone social era, it had put the regulation of the internet back on the agenda, and it had made millions of us reassess our relationship with these companies.

Or had it?

Certainly there seemed to be at least a recognition at Facebook that maybe it had made a few mistakes. Eighteen months after that final report from the DCMS Select Committee I visited the London headquarters of the social media giant, a typically dot.com space with free food at every corner and casually dressed, laptop-toting young employees wandering around having intense conversations. I had come to meet Nicola Mendelsohn, a former advertising executive who had been head of Facebook Europe, and since 2013 its most senior executive outside the United States. We chatted about her own social media history before coming to the company, and how positive just about everyone felt about both Facebook and other tech firms back then. 'There was such a deep love for the brands, for the different tech platforms. Because what they were doing was connecting people in ways that they hadn't been able to connect before.'

So when exactly had that changed? I asked her.

And she gave the same answer I got from Tim Berners-Lee and just about everyone else I interviewed for this book. 'I think it was Cambridge Analytica that really was the key. There were things brewing beforehand, but I think that was a different moment.'

She was in charge by then, and the whole affair had happened in the UK on her watch – so did she feel responsible?

Well, said Mendelsohn,

> I mean, you don't want, with any company that you work at, people to feel angry, disappointed, sad, with what's happened. It was really hard, and of course it was happening in London, but playing out around the world. It was a very challenging time, where lots of things were being thrown at us.

She said they had had to work out what the facts were, and then what to do to rebuild trust, which she admitted would take a long time.

But, sitting there in early 2020, I wondered just how much damage had really been done to Facebook and the people who had led it. Remember, the company stood accused of everything from allowing massive interference in elections to facilitating the persecution of the Rohingya minority in Myanmar. The share price had dived in March 2018 as the Cambridge Analytica story broke and the hashtag #deletefacebook started trending. But on the day I met Nicola Mendelsohn the shares were reaching new highs, valuing the business started in 2004 by Mark Zuckerberg at over $500 billion. While it had become fashionable to insist in the UK and the United States that Facebook had fallen out of favour with the young, it was still growing its audience, which was now approaching 2.5 billion worldwide. Added to this there was Instagram with 1 billion and WhatsApp with 1.6 billion, both owned by Facebook. And while more apologies kept coming, nobody lost their job over the serious breach of trust that had been uncovered in 2018. Chairman and chief executive Mark Zuckerberg, with his special category of shares, had a controlling stake in the business and was not going to relinquish the reins.

The image of Sheryl Sandberg, Zuckerberg's number two and once seen as the kinder, gentler, more human face of the business, had certainly been tarnished by her role in trying to manage the public relations disaster that was the Cambridge Analytica affair. It emerged that Facebook had hired an attack-dog PR firm which had sought to undermine its opponents by stressing their links with the financier and philanthropist George Soros, who was a frequent target for anti-Semitic conspiracy theorists. When it was revealed that, despite earlier denials, the chief operating officer had been copied into emails about the hiring of the firm, it was time for yet another apology. 'Being Jewish is a core part of who I am, and our company stands firmly against hate,' said Sandberg. 'The idea that our work has been interpreted as anti-Semitic is abhorrent to me – and deeply personal.' Still, she and the company weathered the crisis and continued to prosper. But that was not the case for one of those who had fought to expose Facebook's failings.

When I came to meet Damian Collins in Westminster a couple of months after the 2019 General Election, he had just lost his job as chair of the Culture, Media and Sport Select Committee. In the election for the post, he had been defeated by another Conservative backbencher, Julian Knight, who had made it clear that he was far more interested in examining the future of the BBC than continuing to focus on disinformation or the power of the social media giants.

Somehow, Knight had managed to see just about every one of the hundreds of Conservative MPs who were key to the committee election, and there was speculation that Tory whips had facilitated the meetings, keen to manoeuvre the new man into the post. No doubt, after a General Election won on the back of the slogan 'Get Brexit Done', many of the new MPs would have been aware that Damian Collins had clashed repeatedly with Brexiteers as the committee tried to investigate potential Russian interference in the EU referendum. The director of the Vote Leave campaign, Dominic Cummings, had been ruled in contempt of Parliament when he refused to appear in front of the committee, and had told Damian Collins to 'get lost' after he received a summons. Now Cummings, who had himself devised that 'Get Brexit Done' slogan, was the Prime Minister's chief adviser, widely regarded as more powerful than most cabinet ministers. No wonder MPs had been wary of voting for someone seen as an enemy of the new government's chief strategist.

As we sat down in his large, comfortable office in Portcullis House, a legacy of his previous role, Damian Collins was keen to stress that his political career was not over. He would continue to speak out about abuses of power by the tech giants, and he was proud of what the select committee had achieved under his chairmanship.

> Whatever I end up doing in the rest of my working life, I'll always look back on that inquiry and that work and think I made a difference. I think there was a period of time in 2018 where a British parliamentary select committee was probably doing more work than anyone else in the world in scrutinizing some of these issues, which is not normally the case.

I had one last question. Had he left Facebook?

Well, he had deleted the app from his phone, but having a presence was still necessary for his constituency work. For MPs, and for many others, social media had become a vital part of communications infrastructure. You might not like it, you might lament that it meant handing over your data to a few powerful and largely unaccountable corporations on the west coast of the United States, but you could not simply retreat from it.

We can, however, now look back and say that this was the period when the world fell out of love not just with Facebook, but with the whole idea that the smartphone and social media were making our lives better. People who had been worried for some years about the vicious tone of much online discourse, about the hateful behaviour these platforms seemed to enable – cyberbullying, revenge porn, the encouragement of suicide and self-harm – began to wonder if the bad outweighed the good.

I saw this change of mood in two people I had encountered many times over the last 20 years, both of whom had always seemed to embody a huge optimism about what the internet could do for humanity. Jimmy Wales was the founder of the online encyclopedia Wikipedia; Martha Lane Fox had been one of the UK's dot.com pioneers, and had then been appointed by the government to lead efforts to get people online. In the spring of 2020, just as the coronavirus crisis was gathering pace, I had conversations with both of them. Each was at least trying to stay cheerful about the potential of technology to be a force for good.

Jimmy Wales had embraced both smartphones and social media at an early stage and was still an enthusiastic user of Facebook. He had grown up in a small town in Alabama, but he and most of his friends had left when they went to college and never came back. 'A huge proportion of people just scattered. In America, that's very common, and we lost track of each other until Facebook existed.' Now he had reconnected with many of them. They shared good news and bad, and generally kept their friendship ticking over in a way which had not been possible before. 'I've never bought into the criticism of, "Oh, it's all so superficial: we're not really friends any more – we're just Facebook friends." These are my actual friends who I lost touch with, but I appreciate hearing from them.'

But Wales admitted that the belief that in the internet age authoritarian governments could no longer control the flow of information had been naive. China, for instance, had proved it could have a chilling effect on free expression even without plugging every hole in the Great Firewall it had built around the internet. 'The Chinese government doesn't actually believe they can keep educated people from knowing that Liu Xiaobo won the Nobel Peace Prize. But they can certainly keep them from chatting about it.'

Wales had also grown more anxious about the power of the American tech giants, and an advertising-only business model which meant their focus was always to build an audience, keep people engaged, keep them clicking so they could be targeted with more ads. He felt, for instance, that their failure to stop the spread of deranged conspiracy theories or extremist material across their platforms was not deliberate – it was just that the incentives were all wrong.

> I know the people at YouTube and Google very well. I can guarantee you, no one at YouTube ever said, 'Let's try and radicalize young men.' It's just what accidentally happens when you optimize for clicks, for time on site. People are sometimes drawn to ever more radical content because it's fascinating and interesting.

Wales said it was the Cambridge Analytica scandal that had really opened his eyes to the dangers inherent in the targeted advertising business model. And when the ads came in the form of the thousands of targeted messages sent out by the Trump campaign in 2016, that was all the more concerning. 'In the old model of campaign advertising, you still had the sense that a politician had to put out a single consistent narrative that had to appeal to a majority of people. And so you had to persuade people in the middle.' That had all changed with the hyper-targeting that Facebook offered. 'They no longer have to have a single consistent narrative, because they can tell you one thing, and they can tell someone else something else. And that's problematic for democracy.'

Wales contrasted the business model of the social media firms with that of Wikipedia. The online encyclopedia, edited and continuously updated by its own users, has come in for plenty of derision over the years, with critics eager to point out glaring mistakes in some entries, and 'edit wars' breaking out over subjects such as climate change or Donald Trump. But it was by far the most popular reference work on the internet, and a Google search for information on any subject was likely to turn up Wikipedia as its first result. As more people started to ask questions of smart speakers such as the Amazon Echo and the Google Home, it was often Wikipedia which provided the answers. The site was not the place to go if you believed the Earth was flat or that the Moon landings were faked and, while the arguments between editors could become bitter and ideological, the mechanisms for solving disputes seemed to work. Jimmy Wales believes this is

THE WOES OF THE WEB

largely because Wikipedia has never taken advertising, and is mainly funded by donations from well-wishers. 'Our incentives, because of the business model, are never to keep you on the site longer. They're never to give you shareable content, clickbait headlines – you'll never see a clickbait headline in Wikipedia.'

So convinced was the Wikipedia founder that many of the problems of social media and online news were caused by the advertising business model, that he launched a couple of projects that aimed to do things differently. WikiTribune, launched in 2017, was a free news site combining professional journalists with volunteer writers and editors – 'The news is broken. But we figured out how to fix it,' proclaimed its founder. Eighteen months later the paid staff were laid off, though the venture limped on with its volunteers.

In 2019 came another pivot, as Jimmy Wales unveiled WT.Social, a social network which promised quality content with no adverts but supported, like the news site, by voluntary contributions. The argument was that it would be free of the abuse, trolling and misinformation that were staple fare on Facebook and Twitter because, like Wikipedia, it would be policed by the community. That idea seemed attractive, and within days 300,000 people, including me, signed up. But with a plain vanilla website and no phone app, it was not an engaging experience. After a couple of visits I forgot all about it, as I suspect did many others. Taking on Facebook and Instagram, even if millions claimed to be concerned about the way those platforms tracked their users, looked a daunting task.

But when we met, Jimmy Wales refused to admit defeat. 'I'm a pathological optimist,' he said. 'We've had nearly five hundred thousand people sign up. We've got more of them paying than I had hoped for. We're cash flow-positive.'

A couple of weeks later I dropped in on Martha Lane Fox at her West London home and got another dose of optimism, this time about one of the established social media players. Baroness Lane-Fox of Soho – she had been made a peer by David Cameron for her role in getting the UK online – had been a non-executive director of Twitter since 2015. But our meeting had had to be postponed from the previous week because Twitter was in the middle of a crisis.

The social media platform might have become an obsession for millions of people, including both the President of the United States and me, but its growth had stalled, and it was failing to monetize its audience in the way Facebook had. An activist investor group, Elliott Management, was trying to unseat the chief executive Jack Dorsey, unhappy about his strategy and that he had a second job as CEO of the payments firm Square. Martha Lane Fox had been involved in a series of board meetings via video conferencing with San Francisco. But as I arrived that evening the crisis appeared to have passed. Jack Dorsey had met the rebel investors, and they had agreed to work with him in exchange for a seat on the board.

Lane Fox was relieved. She was enthusiastic about Jack Dorsey, and believed he was taking the company in the right direction. Given, however, that she had been a fierce advocate for women who had faced misogynistic abuse online, and that Twitter was struggling to control this and all sorts of other forms of hate speech, conspiracy theories and general trolling, I was curious as to why she still felt so comfortable on the board.

'I really couldn't be in the boardroom if I didn't think that the direction of travel was positive, not negative for Twitter,' she explained. 'You might disagree with my own personal choice, but what I perceive is that Twitter is fundamentally structured around some things that I think are right.' She talked about it being open rather than closed, about its role in improving the quality of general conversation. She admitted that the firm had been slow to react to the abuse of high-profile women on its platform. 'But is that getting any better? Yes, it's vastly better. Look at their safety and abuse reports, and the amount of reports are dramatically down.'

Then I brought up Donald Trump, who used Twitter to bully and belittle everyone from his political opponents to any journalist who dared question him. Surely that was not 'improving the quality of conversation?'

She pushed back hard. 'I don't buy that argument. Sure, if he does stuff that contravenes the policies, he should be treated like any other user, but, you know, this notion that somehow Trump has his platform just through Twitter – crap. I mean, absolute crap!' Trump had far fewer followers than his predecessor Barack Obama, she pointed out, but traditional media organizations, including the BBC, chose to amplify his tweets. Later, of course, Twitter did decide to remove Trump's megaphone.

While Lane Fox largely exonerated Twitter, she did, however, concede that the whole mood about the nature of the Web and digital technology had darkened, even before the Cambridge Analytica scandal.

> Five years ago, it feels to me, the shine was coming off in people's minds about technology platforms, full stop. In my opinion, it's a conflagration of lots of things: not paying taxes, American conglomerates, globalization, what's happening with my own data.

But what happened in 2016 crystallized that darker mood, she said, comparing it to a fairground game. 'It's like one of those things in the arcade when all the pennies move, and then a couple of pennies fall, and the whole thing falls over the edge. The thing that maybe tipped it was the Cambridge Analytica stuff, plus Trump, plus Brexit, plus general anxiety.'

Despite it all, Martha Lane Fox too remained a determined optimist. She had lived through the ups and downs of the first dot.com bubble. Then in 2004 she had been in a car crash in Morocco which very nearly killed her and kept her in hospital for two years. She had emerged just as smartphones and social media were taking off, and had embraced both with huge enthusiasm. 'I remember with the iPhone thinking, oh, wow! this is transformational! – because even though I was quite broken I could really do a lot of stuff.' She had joined the board of Marks and Spencer, and kept on evangelizing about how the smartphone would transform the way people shopped – to the bemusement of many of her fellow directors. As for Facebook, 'it was a great way to keep up with the nurses that looked after me in hospital.' Then she had moved over to Twitter, finding it was full of the kind of interesting techie people she needed to know in her role as Gordon Brown's Digital Champion. 'It was phenomenal for me in building up a network of people who knew what they were talking about in terms of helping people get digital skills.'

And in 2020, at a particularly dark time, when a global pandemic was under way, Lane Fox still thought the technology which she had helped persuade millions of Britons to adopt was a positive force. It wound her up, she told me, when journalists asked her why she still wanted to broaden access to the internet now we knew about its perils – 'those people still do their shopping online every week!' For all its downsides, the smartphone era had given people all sorts of tools that were enriching their lives.

But a few weeks earlier the Web's creator, the man who had fired the starting gun for the online era, had not seemed so sanguine. In a video-conference call to his Boston home, I asked Sir Tim Berners-Lee when he had first suspected that his creation was going wrong.

He admitted that for many years he had brushed off many of the concerns. He visited the bits of the Web he liked, not those he did not. 'When people came to me and said, "I found something horrible on the Web," I would say, "Well, that's your fault, because you followed links. Wherever you followed it from, don't do it again."' But he said what had happened in 2016 'with Trump and Brexit' had been a wake-up call. He had realized that he and his friends were living in one filter bubble, but millions were living in another: one which had been 'deliberately and maliciously created by criminal and foreign forces'.

Hitherto he had thought that if people behaved badly to one another online, or spread untruths about climate change or other issues he cared about, that just did not affect him. But then he came to a sudden realization: 'Those people *vote*. Why should I worry about it? The answer is that, actually, they live in the same country, and they *vote*.'

Berners-Lee's vision of the Web as a borderless, open, liberal community, free from censorship and any kind of government control, was fading. The Web was indeed 'for everyone', as he had put it in his message during the Olympics' opening ceremony – but that everyone included crooks, conspiracy theorists and millions who simply did not share the values of a liberal, middle-aged English scientist.

We may have begun to feel more dubious about the computers in our pockets. But we're all still carrying them around with us – unable to resist peeking at the latest Trump tweet, playing games, watching videos and a hundred other things.

What is that doing to our heads?

8

Always On

We carry them with us wherever we go, we look at them hundreds of times a day, and we panic every time we cannot find them or realize we left them at home. But how often do we think about what our smartphones know about *us*, and what we are telling the giant tech companies as we use their various services on the move? And given how central they have become to our lives, should we worry about how healthy our relationship with our phones is? These are questions I asked of just about every person I met for this book and, as I went on this voyage of discovery in the UK and in California, I began to find out about my own intimate and perhaps addictive relationship with my phone.

On a spring day in 2020 I went in search of expert analysis of the modern smartphone and what it could do. Some months later, as I sat down to write this, I could recreate that day by looking back at the data my phone generated. My photo collection, for instance, told me exactly where I was at 06.41 that morning: in the park walking the dog. The next picture was labelled Ealing Broadway Station, with the timestamp 08.52. It showed me sitting on a Central Line Tube train waiting for it to depart, and grabbing a sneaky picture of the woman sitting opposite me. Why? Because she was wearing a face mask which, a couple of weeks before the coronavirus pandemic brought the UK to a halt, was still an unusual sight. Looking through my sent emails on the phone, I could see that I messaged a colleague about a story I was chasing before the train disappeared underground.

The Google Maps app records every location you visit, and your iPhone also keeps a list of recent locations. So I could see that on that day I went first to my office in central London, then on to my appointment. The payments app told me I stopped to buy a coffee on the way. My destination was clear from the next photo: skyscrapers against a blue sky in a Canary Wharf office development at 10.52. A few minutes later there was another picture – of a bottle of hand sanitiser at the reception desk of the company I was visiting. Again, this was still unusual enough in those innocent days to merit a photo.

I had come to see James Chappell, co-founder and chief technology officer of Digital Shadows. His company was founded to help organizations cope with the security challenges of a new world in which everyone had started bringing their own devices to work. 'We saw a lot of security people saying businesses can't engage with social media, they can't engage in mobile apps, because the sky will fall and that'll be the end of humanity as we know it,' he explained. 'But the reality was that they didn't have a choice: they were being outpaced by their competitors who were adopting digital technology.'

So Chappell set about advising on the safe use of these devices, which meant understanding exactly what kind of data they were collecting and sharing. He looked at my iPhone and began to count the different ways it monitored me. 'Pretty much all iPhones have some sort of barometric pressure reader, so I can tell what altitude someone is at, velocity sensors so I can tell when you're awake or when you're asleep.' If your phone is not moving and it's the middle of the night, that is a pretty good clue that you're asleep. Many people then pick up their phone the moment they wake.

Chappell counted at least five types of radio communication on my phone. 'There is Bluetooth, Wi-Fi, two types of cellular radio – one for voice, another for data – and then on my phone and many like it there is NFC, Near Field Communications, allowing applications such as Apple Pay. So that's all giving quite a rich set of data.'

Then there were more sensors, an accelerometer measuring how fast the phone is moving, a compass, multiple cameras – no fewer than four on my phone . . . 'And light sensors, so depending on whether I'm holding it up to my ear or away from my face you can tell whether it's light or dark.' And James realized he had missed another radio system, GPS, which told the phone where it was. In summary, these devices are collecting a vast amount of information.

So who has access to it? Well, the phone maker and the network operators have some of it, and then there is what we allow app developers to know about us. Every time we installed an app, James explained, we were asked to decide, for instance, whether it should be allowed to know where we were, or to access the phone's camera or microphone. 'As a consumer you want to feel that you're entering into some kind of transaction, that you're in theory deciding to trade some of that data in exchange for some value.' He gave as an example a measurement app he had installed on his phone which he used when visiting a builder's merchant to buy some timber. The app was free but supported by adverts and, as he put it, 'if you're not paying for something you're the product.' He was handing over data about his location and the kind of goods he bought so that the app developer could provide advertisers with that information. They would then be able to target him better. 'They know I was in Camden Town, they know I was buying building materials. They've got access to a bunch of data to help them be more effective in making money, monetising that free user base. I'm fine with that. I don't have a problem as a consumer.'

This advertising model, based on user data, is how much of the internet works. 'Data is the new oil' has become a tired cliché, but for online advertising giants it has proved true: Google and Facebook have become the Standard Oil or BP of the digital era, reaping vast profits from their access to our data, most of it now from our mobile phones.

For a while, back in 2012 as it prepared to launch its shares on the New York Stock Exchange, Facebook appeared concerned that it would not adapt to the smartphone era. When the company published the official document giving details of its forthcoming Initial Public Offering, it listed 35 risks to its future. Here is how number 3 on that list read: 'Growth in use of Facebook through our mobile products, where our ability to monetize is unproven, as a substitute for use on personal computers may negatively affect our revenue and financial results.' It need not have worried. Within a couple of years Facebook had proved that it could 'monetize' us on our phones, and by 2018 92 per cent of its advertising revenues were coming from mobile, generating over $50 billion annually.

James Chappell said he was careful about the permissions he gave to app developers like Facebook, and in general was pretty relaxed about this bargain where he handed over some data in exchange for a free service. But there was one new area of mobile phone data collection that did worry him: information about people's faces. 'If you think of the number of faces you collect, either on your mobile device or in your social media – those faces become available quite often in the public domain.' Not only are many phones using your face to identify you when you log on, but we are also all helping to build a massive facial recognition database every time we tag a photo on a social media platform.

Just how powerful that kind of database could be emerged when the *New York Times* revealed in 2020 that a small company called Clearview AI had scraped billions of photos from social media to build a facial recognition app which US police forces were using to identify suspects. Facebook, YouTube and Twitter sent cease-and-desist letters to the company, and the police forces said they would stop using the app. But James Chappell said the incident had shown that the genie was out of the bottle. In countries with more relaxed views of privacy there was nothing to stop another organization or perhaps a government doing the same thing. 'The social media companies would be exceptionally annoyed, and they actually work very hard to put in place controls to stop third parties from doing this. But if they want the data enough they're going to get it.'

I left the offices of Digital Shadows with a new awareness that I was carrying with me a powerful surveillance device. Of course, some of the data my phone was collecting was for my benefit. The Health app on my phone, coupled with my smartwatch, tells me all about how active I have been, and on that day I had done well. I had exercised for

108 minutes, walking the dog and making my way around London for various appointments, and that meant I had burned through 1,006 calories, well above my 750-calorie target. But a relatively new feature of my phone told a more worrying story about my lifestyle.

In 2018 Apple had introduced something called ScreenTime, a log of your daily activity on your phone. Like other technology firms, Apple had been accused of making its products addictive, so this new feature was promoted as part of a digital wellbeing initiative. The app not only recorded how long you had spent looking at your phone and what activities occupied most time, it allowed you to set limits, either for yourself or for children whose devices you controlled. That day, the ScreenTime app showed I had spent 8 hours and 2 minutes on my phone, with more than half of that on social media sites. For 3 hours and 17 minutes I had been sucked in by Twitter – no surprise to my wife, who had long accused me of being a Twitterholic. The app also counted 171 'pick-ups' – times I had picked up my phone – and most of them were to check Twitter. Then the many apps and news sources I had signed up to receive had sent me 107 notifications. In other words, an information avalanche was reaching me via my smartphone, and I in turn was contributing to other people's flood of data with my constant tweets, Facebook posts, WhatsApp messages and emails.

I activated ScreenTime as soon as it became available, and every Sunday I got sent a report showing my week's data, and whether it had risen or fallen. I cannot say that this made me change my behaviour, and I did not take advantage of the tool which allows you to limit your screen time with enforced breaks. But the arrival of this and similar monitoring apps for Android was a marker that there was something of a moral panic under way about the impact of smartphones, and in particular whether they were harming the mental health of children.

Towards the end of the 2010s, a number of articles, some from academics, others from less qualified pundits, sounded the alarm about an impending mental health crisis threatening the children of the smartphone era. Perhaps the most influential appeared in the *Atlantic*, a very sober literary and cultural magazine, and as far from a shock-horror tabloid as you can imagine. The headline in the September 2017 edition of the magazine read, 'Have Smartphones Destroyed A Generation?' and the author was Jean Twenge, a professor of psychology at San Diego State University. She described the habits of what she called iGen, young people born between 1995 and 2012. They were 'growing up with smartphones, have an Instagram account before they start high school, and do not remember a time before the internet.'

These young people were physically safer than previous generations – they were involved in fewer car accidents and drank less – but were on the brink of the 'worst mental health crisis in decades', with much of the deterioration being the fault of their smartphones. They were spending less time dating, fewer of them were having sex, and having a part-time job doing a paper round or working in a supermarket was going out of fashion. What they were doing far more of was sitting in their rooms looking at their phones.

Data from an annual survey of teenagers showed, said Professor Twenge, there was a correlation between excessive screen use and depression. 'The results could not be clearer: teens who spend more time than average on screen activities are more likely to be unhappy.' The article painted a picture of a lonely and depressed generation, looking at social media first thing in the morning and last thing at night, afflicted by sleeplessness and even suicidal thoughts.

As we will find out later, not every academic thought Jean Twenge's analysis stood up to scrutiny. But it fed into a wider concern that parents might be sleepwalking into a crisis which could cause serious damage to their children.

In the UK, one person who frequently contacted me to express such concerns was a marketing consultant called Belinda Parmar. I first met Belinda more than a decade ago when she set up an organization called Lady Geek to encourage more women to take an interest in technology, and help companies market to them better. She had been infuriated by the extraordinarily sexist assumptions made by tech firms – an electronics retailer running a campaign with the slogan 'My world is pink'; a computer maker creating a portal for women which offered them recipes alongside technology advice. As well as being an adept campaigner, she was a great voice to include in technology reports at a time when just about all of the pundits seemed to be men. She was of course an enthusiastic early adopter of smartphones and social media and, looking back, said she could not have built her business without one particular site: 'Twitter was an amazing way to get my ideas out to an already interested population of geeks, and non-geeks,' she told me when I spoke to her in 2020.

But gradually she had turned against technology. She explained that she realized now that she had been so absorbed in her phone that she was neglecting her small children. 'I remember checking my Twitter feed before checking on my kids.' She had come to see her phone and the constant social media updates as a kind of drug: 'It tapped into my insecurities, all of our insecurities – I need that validation, I need to feel that we belong. I need to feed my ego. And that's my worry with smartphones: that they actually tapped into our anxiety.' Belinda was convinced that the companies behind these devices were engineering them to make them addictive. 'For every one of us trying to not look at our screen, there are thousands of developers, designers, psychologists who are playing mind monopoly with us.'

But it was the impact of these technologies on children rather than adults that was her main worry. She began campaigning about the dangers after a friend's son became so obsessed with video games that he became the first person in the UK to be diagnosed with games addiction. As she spoke to me down a video-conferencing connection, Belinda told me that we were sleepwalking into a mental health crisis, with smartphones and other screens trapping children in their bedrooms and stopping them from having healthy interactions with the real world. I pressed her on what evidence there was of teenagers coming to harm. She reeled off facts from a number of studies – one looked at 23,000 adults and found that excessive screen time correlated with poor mental health; another found that girls who spent over three hours a day on social media were twice as likely to suffer with depression.

I put it to her that a recent report from Britain's Royal College of Paediatricians had found there was little evidence that the use of screens by children was harmful in itself, although it said they should be avoided for the hour before bedtime.

She snorted, and told me that in a television discussion she had confronted one of the study's authors. 'I said, have you spent any time with teenagers in the last eighteen months?' Belinda brushed aside my suggestion that we just had insufficient data to reach firm conclusions about the impact of screen use. 'Of course we don't, but that is because it's so new. But we just need to spend time with some teenagers to worry about the empathy levels, and the ability to socialize, and the addiction. I think it's there – we don't want to see it.'

Over the ages there have been moral panics about every new communication technology, from the telegraph to radio to television. Hadn't parents once feared that TV was turning their children into zombies? I asked.

'The TV didn't show you content that was inappropriate for your age,' she said. 'The TV is in a public place where your parents or guardians have access to it. And the TV is a passive experience, and doesn't give you the same level of dopamine.'

It seemed strange that someone whose whole mission had been about evangelizing the benefits of technology should have turned against it with such venom. But she had put some of her thinking into a new direction in her work, moving on from Lady Geek to a consultancy she called the Empathy Business.

Major companies such as Centrica and Barclays were hiring her to bring more empathy into their organizations. She said her aim was to transform their way of work and 'rehumanize' it. She was not working with major technology companies, but she had strong words for them. She had been furious to hear the chief executive of Netflix, Reed Hastings, say that his company's main rival for customer attention was not YouTube or the broadcasters, but people's need to sleep. 'Responsible leadership is not putting in pool tables and giving people free smoothies. Responsible leadership is thinking about the vulnerability and protection of our children. And, yes, you can make money – but at the same time you have to do good and you have to have a purpose.'

While not everyone was as convinced as Belinda Parmar that technology was rotting our children's brains, there had been a substantial backlash against the tech giants and the 'move fast and break things' culture of Silicon Valley. And, a decade after the launch of the addictive iPhone, it seemed even technology executives were becoming wary of letting their own children spend too much time glued to gadgets, and were also becoming more concerned about their own 'always on' lifestyles. Mindfulness was the new trend and, in typical Silicon Valley fashion, entrepreneurs soon realized there was a huge business opportunity in addressing the very problems that the technology had helped to create.

Among them was Michael Acton Smith, the British founder of a number of companies, from the online gadget retailer Firebox to MindCandy, maker of the children's game Moshi Monsters. That business had made him one of the best-known figures on the UK tech scene, a tousle-haired party animal who somehow managed to be both hip and establishment, and had been awarded an OBE in 2014 for services to the creative industries.

Lauded as one of Britain's fastest growing companies, MindCandy was said to be on the verge of an IPO that would reap a huge pay-out for its founder. But in the smartphone era its fortunes faded. Moshi Monsters, Smith admits, never really adapted to the rapid move from the web to mobile. 'I didn't fully appreciate how enormous the shift was going to be,' he told me in early 2020. 'I think we were a little late to recognize just how huge.'

Acton Smith could afford to be philosophical about the fact that the business had never quite achieved the success that had seemed within its grasp. After all, we were talking in the spacious downtown San Francisco offices of his new, fast-growing company. There were all the accoutrements we have come to expect of a tech office: free food, outsized pot plants, and a mission statement emblazoned on a wall: 'To make the world healthier and happier.'

This was the headquarters of Calm, a mindfulness and meditation app that had achieved unicorn status – in other words, it had been valued at over a billion dollars while still a private company.

The company had been launched in London in 2012 with another British entrepreneur Alex Tew as co-founder. Tew had made his name back in 2005 with an ingenious idea to pay his way through university, the Million Dollar Homepage, where he charged $1 per pixel for advertising space on a giant web page. He and Michael had shared a house in London and had both practised meditation for years. Michael said they had spotted the opportunity presented by an ever more stressful, technology-driven world:

> We just had an inkling, an entrepreneur's kind of sixth sense that this was coming, and that it was only going to continue. The world was not going to be getting any less stressful. We were not going to be spending less time on our devices and our computers. And therefore, anxiety would be increasing, stress would be increasing, depression would be increasing, all the other mental health issues would be growing.

They soon decided that Silicon Valley was the place to grow their business. 'We felt that a business like Calm should be based in California,' Michael told me. 'People were just more receptive and open to mindfulness than they were in London, and then, connected to that, I think we felt it would just be a better place to raise capital.'

It certainly was. An app that promised to reduce stress, help you sleep and build self-esteem – something not in short supply in California – won a big audience, with 40 million downloads and a million subscribers, gaining the attention of some of the most influential venture capitalists. In February 2019 it had raised another $88 million for expansion at a valuation of $1 billion, becoming the world's first mental health unicorn.

When I visited that chilled-out San Francisco office a year later, the good times were still rolling. Michael was just back from a week in Los Angeles, where he had been recruiting new staff and discussing possible celebrity endorsements for the app. Already the actor Matthew McConaughey and the writer and actor Stephen Fry were working with Calm, lending their soothing voices to the bedtime stories which, along with whalesong, were among the app's standout features. The mood in the office seemed busy but, well, calm – just like its founder.

But I wanted to explore the paradoxes in Michael Acton Smith's life and this business. Here was someone who had spent two decades at the very intense frontline of the tech start-up world, a place where rivalries were fierce, work/life balance was a joke and, in the words of the Intel founder Andy Grove, only the paranoid survive. Yet here he was preaching a message that we all needed to chill out, have a more balanced attitude to work, maybe put down our gadgets – well, apart from our smartphones with our Calm app – and think about what was really important in life.

I was keen to know whether that also applied to the staff working around us – and to the way he now lived. He smiled, and said he accepted that there was a paradox, but that they tried to make sure that people could work from home, and the whole emphasis of the business was not about moving fast and breaking things but on responsible growth. 'We're very ambitious,' he admitted. 'We want to build one of the most valuable and meaningful companies in the world. And we can't do that just by working nine to five.' He said rather than a work/life balance, he preferred to talk of a work/life blend:

> Work can be incredibly challenging and exciting and rewarding. We don't want to burn people out and have them working around the clock – the 9–9–6 that we hear about in China, which is 9 a.m. to 9 p.m. six days a week, is absolutely not what we want to do here. But we want to work with people who are stimulated by their work and want to make a difference in the world.

We moved on to his take on what smartphones have done to us. He called them 'magic boxes – some of the wonders of the world; one of the most extraordinary technologies ever built.' But then, in language surprisingly like that I had heard from Belinda Parmar, he suggested there was a problem: not with the technology but how we used it. 'Most of us use these incredibly powerful devices in a mindless way. We're like dopamine-frazzled zombies, just looping through looking for those hits.'

Ah, but of course there was a solution. *We all needed to practise mindfulness.* 'When you change your relationship to your device, if you have a more mindful relationship, if you build up a meditation practice, you can use your devices and technology to help your life rather than hinder it. And I think that changes everything.' He said he practised this himself and had become more 'mindful' of how he used his phone. He did not take it to bed, and left it in airplane mode until he left home in the morning in order to stem the constant flow of news and notifications.

> I think the majority of people, when they wake up, the first thing they do is reach for their phone, and as soon as you're checking Twitter and Instagram and the news your brain is just into those loops. And I think it's really valuable to have half an hour or an hour in the morning without marinating your brain in the digital minutiae of the world.

Michael Acton Smith was not alone in being concerned about the impact smartphones were having on his well-being. Just about everybody I met for this book seemed to have decided they needed to limit either their own or their children's screen time. The Wikipedia founder Jimmy Wales, another huge optimist about the impact of these technologies in general, admitted that the problem in his household was more about the parents than their children: 'I do remember once our little girl said to us on vacation, "Can we just have one meal please without Mommy being on the phone?"' He put some of the blame on the way smartphones and social media were designed.

I think a lot of the technologies are in some cases – I think accidentally – designed to be addictive. If you think about an algorithm to keep people on the site as long as possible in order to show them as many ads as possible, that means it's going to be addictive, and it's going to be designed for certain kinds of stimuli. Once you've got an advertising medium, on the devices in your hand or in your pocket 24 hours a day, it's going to be designed in a way that's potentially problematic.

The dot.com entrepreneur and UK internet advocate Martha Lane Fox admitted she was slightly addicted to her smartphone, in particular measuring her steps on it, which she described as 'ridiculous and pointless'. But she said she never took her phone into her bedroom, and did not have notifications set up. She also felt that people like her who had started tech firms in the late 1990s had long been used to being always on – 'having to be by my email because there was going to be some customer service collapse at [her company] lastminute.com if I wasn't' – and had not been particularly concerned about it until they had children. 'That generation's anxiety came when they saw their children completely aping the behaviour of their parents when they were on their smartphones. It felt like an inflection point: lots of the tech crowd in the UK suddenly having kids, and suddenly getting anxious about it.'

Even the man who first brought the iPhone to the UK was getting anxious in 2020 about some of the impact it was having. Sir Charles Dunstone, founder of Carphone Warehouse, said that overall there were all sorts of positive changes in society caused by smartphones and social media – 'you create communities not limited by proximity.' That also gave people far more power as consumers, cutting out intermediaries and making life a lot tougher for businesses. But he also felt too many people were captured by their phones. 'You get to Euston Station and there's just a whole lot of zombies, walking around looking at this thing in front of them, and as a result we don't see the people in the world around us.'

I asked him what his phone told him about his own screen time.

'Four hours and nine minutes a day: twenty per cent down on last week.'

Nothing like as bad as mine, I told him.

But again, he was worried about his children's screen habits. 'My kids are still quite young, but they are obsessed with them, and it's now a battle. If you're not careful, they don't want to play outside or ride a bike or do anything.'

Even among the very people who had brought us this technology revolution, then, there was a degree of anxiety about how it was changing our lives. But much of what they described about changing behaviour was impressionistic and anecdotal. I wanted to know what hard data there might be about the effects of screen time. And even if those I'd consulted were mostly optimistic about the technology, they were all middle-aged, rather than digital natives who had never known anything different.

I decided I needed to speak to two more people: a young person who had grown up with smartphones, and an academic who had a good overview of the data about screen use. Luckily, I found one person to do both jobs. Dr Amy Orben is an experimental psychologist who is a research fellow at Cambridge University's MRC Cognition and Brain Sciences Unit.

I met her in a crowded London café on a chilly winter's day. It was noisy, and I was worried that the voice transcription app on my smartphone that I now use for all of my interviews would not pick up what she said. But so precisely did she speak – and so smart was the machine learning in the app – that her voice and the transcript came through loud and clear when I checked it afterwards.

I began by asking what she remembered about the iPhone launch back in 2007. 'I was thirteen,' she said. 'I don't really remember the iPhone being unveiled.'

(On the recording you can hear me saying 'Oh my God!' as I realize quite how young that made this woman who had already got her doctorate and a Cambridge fellowship.)

Amy, whose parents are German, spent her childhood partly in New York, partly in Germany, in what she described as 'a pretty tech-sceptic household'. In New York she attended a very traditional school – 'I think the parents needed to agree not to let the kids watch TV at home' – so it was a while before she got a smartphone. 'I got an iPhone 3, the one with the rounded edges, I think probably at the end of my school days in 2010.' She remembered the craze among her school friends for the Blackberry and the BBM messaging system, and then joining Facebook around the same time. 'I mainly used it for quizzes – you know, what Disney Princess are you?' Then she went to Cambridge as an undergraduate to study psychology, right at the moment when the use of smartphones and social media by students was at its most intense. 'People would go on a night out and take, like, a hundred crappy pictures and upload the hundred crappy pictures to Facebook,' she remembered.

I asked what she had thought about that.

'I think as an undergrad, it's all about exploring who you are, and being seen, and showing that you have friends, and so it was really normal at the time.'

But soon, as well as plunging into social media as a key part of student life, Amy was taking a professional interest in Facebook. She noticed the acquisition of Instagram and then WhatsApp, and realized how powerful a role the company now had. 'Suddenly I was, like, wow! They're doing their job really well, because this is all the communication I'd ever need . . .'

By 2015 she was doing her undergraduate dissertation on Facebook personality data. This, remember, was around the time that a Cambridge University psychologist, Aleksandr Kogan, was harvesting data from a Facebook personality quiz. Amy remembers attending a couple of Kogan's social psychology lectures, and met him once when she was trying to work out a subject for a summer project. She looked around the Web for the research that was being done into social media by academics who, unlike her, were not digital natives. She was not impressed.

I felt like a lot of the research being done didn't speak to my experience using social media. They had no clue what was going on. You'd read things like, 'People go on Facebook to make new friends,' and you'd think I've never made a new friend. I was amazed at how rudimentary the work was.

She was convinced she could do better, and started work on a doctorate looking at the way in which social media was changing the way we form social connections.

Then the Cambridge Analytica scandal broke, and getting hold of Facebook data even for respectable academic research became virtually impossible. She switched her focus to the impact of screen time on teenagers, which was, as we've seen, becoming a hot new area – perhaps because it was easier to get access to data. Once again, she found the quality of research in this area disappointing. It was the work of Professor Jean Twenge, author of the seminal *Atlantic* article, that really caught her eye. Since then Twenge's book *i-Gen* had been published, again warning about the dire impact of smartphones on the mental health of American teenagers. Then there was a report from the Royal Society for Public Health, which rated social media platforms for their impact on mental health. It found that YouTube was the most positive, while Instagram and Snapchat came bottom in terms of their detrimental effect on the mental health of young people. This was based on a questionnaire in which teenagers were asked to rank the different platforms in areas such as their impact on sleep, self-esteem, loneliness and depression.

'I was kind of horrified by the quality of the research,' said Amy. She later took it apart in a lengthy blogpost. Her argument was that using a questionnaire asking teenagers to give single answers about how they felt various social media platforms affected their anxiety levels, or the way they slept, was a hopelessly flawed technique. Moreover, the research had been marketed to the media and garnered lurid headlines before it had even been peer-reviewed. 'Does the public health charity care more about their media coverage than about correctly informing the public?' she asked. What was needed were long-term studies that measured real mental health outcomes, such as whether somebody had been diagnosed with depression.

This was a 22-year-old academic right at the start of her career taking on an august body – almost the definition of chutzpah. But Amy was not finished. It was the Jean Twenge book and a subsequent academic paper that was now in her crosshairs. 'I got so annoyed that I started writing to editors, I posted tirades on Twitter,' she remembered. Once again, she was taking on someone older and much more experienced – this time a professor of psychology at San Diego State University, and the author, according to her website, 'of more than 130 scientific publications and six books.'

iGen, the book that had caused such a stir, had been published before the research on which she based it appeared in academic journals. Amy's main concern, she told me, was that Jean Twenge's conclusions about the harmful effects of smartphones appeared to be a case of 'correlation is not causation.' Sure, you might find data that said there was a rise in teenage depression which began about the time the iPhone was launched, but that did not mean that one led to the other. Amy did not dispute that there was some evidence linking smartphones and social media to a decline in mental health. She just thought it was pretty sketchy. Or, as she later put it in an academic paper reviewing the state of research into this subject: 'The association between digital technology use, or social media use in particular, and psychological well-being is – on average – negative but very small.' What's more, you could not be sure whether it was excessive screen use which led to poor mental health, or poor mental health which led to excessive screen use. 'The direction of the link between digital technology use and well-being is still unclear: effects have been found to exist in both directions and there has been little work done to rule out potential confounders.'

As we sat in a café where most people seemed to be staring at their phones I brought up the issue of addiction – wasn't that a thing?

Amy grimaced. 'It's like I say I'm addicted to cheese, I'm addicted to fries, I'm addicted to chocolate. I would also say I'm addicted to my phone.' But she said addiction had a clinical meaning for an academic. 'It's something that has lifelong consequences, causes clinical changes in the brain. So we need to be incredibly cautious in saying social media addiction is a thing.'

Back in 2017, this whole debate, and the annoyance Amy felt at seeing what she regarded as low-quality research getting big headlines, had a profound effect on the direction of her life. She had been heading out of academia, interviewing for jobs as a management consultant. Instead, she seems to have been energized by her clashes with the merchants of smartphone doom, seeing a new path for her research.

As her own media profile rose, she was invited to take part in an hour-long debate on the BBC World Service with a catchy headline – 'Are Smartphones Harming Teenagers?' It was her first appearance on the radio and she was a little nervous – and even more so when the producer told her that one of the other guests was Professor Jean Twenge.

As the recording got under way, Twenge stressed that she had been in this field for more than 25 years, and had examined large amounts of data about the mental health of American teenagers. She talked of a 50 per cent increase in rates of depression, a doubling and then tripling of the suicide rate, and quoted studies which said social media use led to depression rather than the other way round. 'You can't, of course, say definitively, OK, we know for sure it's smartphones,' she said. 'But there's a lot pointing in this direction.'

The presenter introduced Amy, making the point that at 22 she was perhaps part of the 'iGen' generation described by Jean Twenge. She picked up and ran with this idea. 'I think coming from both the younger generation, and researching social media gives me additional insight.' She took on the much more experienced academic, challenging her data on mental health and questioning the causal link with smartphones, and came up with a startling example of why correlation does not equal causation:

Just because two things happen at the same time, doesn't mean that they cause each other. For example, I looked around a bit this morning trying to find other things that correlate with each other.

And I found that suicides by hanging correlates to 99.8 per cent with the US spending for science, space and technology.

Jean Twenge fired back, pointing out that when the deterioration in teenagers' mental health happened between 2011 and 2015, the biggest change was them spending more time on their smartphones, and less time away from screens doing things like interacting with their friends in person.

The young researcher and the more experienced academic agreed that there was a need for more data, though Jean Twenge insisted that action on this urgent issue could not wait. But when Amy suggested this could be just another moral panic like that around video games earlier, which had proved to be wrong, Professor Twenge intervened down the line from Florida. 'I disagree with that completely, given the meta-analyses!'

Hardly a meeting of minds, then, and I suspect most listeners to the programme came away with an uneasy feeling that there was an issue, and maybe they should be worried about teenagers being glued to their smartphones. But Amy told me she came out of the studio really happy. 'I had all the points I wanted to make written down and I was crossing them off.' She became the go-to dissident voice in the debate on the evils of smartphones. 'It was crazy – I was on *Woman's Hour*, on the *Today* programme, and I got ripped apart by Jeremy Vine,' she told me gleefully. She also gave evidence to the House of Commons Science and Technology Select Committee and got involved in reports on screen time by a number of professional organisations. Here she felt she did have an impact: most of the reports ended up saying there was not yet enough evidence to reach the scary conclusions about the effects of this pervasive technology that people like Belinda Parmar and Jean Twenge had been airing.

Perhaps the moral panic was fading. But Amy did not just walk away. She plunged deeper into her research on the effects of smartphones and social media on well-being. She had concluded that academics had been going down the wrong path:

I think we didn't find any results because we were asking a way too general question. Asking whether screen time is good or bad for kids is for me like asking, is eating sugar good or bad for kids? Well, if your child is a severe diabetic, eating that chocolate bar might kill them. But if they just came off the football pitch it might be really helpful.

The young people who owned smartphones came from all sorts of backgrounds and they used them in all sorts of diverse ways – they might be watching porn, playing a violent video game or reading Shakespeare for a homework assignment. The research needed to reflect that diversity. As with many areas of life, Amy Orben had decided that the answer to whether too much screen time was bad for you was . . . it's complicated.

After our meeting early in 2020, the arrival of the coronavirus pandemic saw Dr Orben embark on new research into how young people turned to technology during lockdowns. Her initial findings were that smartphones and other screens were proving their worth, whether it was helping young people to continue their education or allowing them to keep in touch with friends and family. In November 2020 she told me that the virus had shown how lazy the assumption of many policymakers was that time spent looking at screens was wasted – the 'Why don't you go outside and do something useful?' argument.

'Lockdown really challenged that idea, and it needed to be challenged,' she says. 'For example, for certain disadvantaged groups it might be a really important way of getting information and getting in contact with people like you – for instance if you're an LGBTQ teen in a very small town.'

So how did I emerge from my encounters with these differing viewpoints on the impact of being 'always on'?

Well, on the one hand I remained naturally sceptical about the kind of moral panics that Amy Orben describes. From the novel to video games, from the telegraph to television, society has greeted every new technology with anxiety about its impact on everything from teenage pregnancies to church attendance. What's more, the impact of smartphones on my ability to connect with people both personally and professionally has been mostly enriching – and, as we will find out later, you would not want to be without one during a global pandemic.

But I did have concerns about the obsessive nature of these devices: the way they lured you away from whatever you should be doing. While writing these last few paragraphs, for instance, I picked up my phone half a dozen times to check a tweet or a text, until I eventually took it downstairs to stop it being a distraction.

And then there is the technology industry, and the vast army of public relations and marketing executives all pushing the message that the very latest gizmo is essential to your health, wealth and happiness. After more than two decades dealing with the hucksters and hype merchants of this industry I may have grown just a little cynical.

9

Spinners, Hacks and Hype

On a typical day, something like 300 emails come piling into my BBC inbox, many of them from public relations executives with a story to sell about some amazing innovation. Back in 2014, figures from the US Department of Labor showed there were 4.6 PRs to every journalist, and I am sure that number must have since grown, especially when it comes to those employed to promote technology companies.

I have just typed the words 'extraordinary', 'exciting', 'revolutionary' and 'VIP' into the search box of Microsoft Outlook to see what comes up. '**Extraordinary** Opportunity to Experience the World's 6G Hotspot Followed by the World's First Open 5G Cyber Security Hackathon in Oulu, Finland', reads one email. Then there is news of 'a **revolutionary** new laser-marking technique to address tampering and counterfeiting in diamonds'. The PR man for a mobile phone company is excited: 'Hi Rory, Properly **exciting** news from OnePlus today'. The marketing folks behind the 'self-driving hub Zenzic' would love me to come to a private breakfast (rather than a public one, you understand) 'to hear an **exciting** announcement on its Connected and Automated Mobility (CAM) Roadmap to 2030'. And then there's a '**VIP** Press Invitation to 2020 Crypto Briefing Brunch'. It is always extraordinary, exciting, even revolutionary to find out that a humble technology reporter is a VIP, even if I would not attend a crypto briefing brunch in a thousand years – and in any case that event, like just about everything in 2020, was cancelled.

Many of these messages get only a cursory glance – but the most diligent PRs are not deterred by a failure to respond. 'I'm just checking in to see if you received my previous email pitch . . . The topic suggested was: How to solve the problem of cryptocurrency volatility.' And then those who have 'reached out' and failed to get a reply have another useful bit of jargon in their armoury: 'Circling back on my invitation from last week . . .' 'Just circling back to see if you have any interest in . . .' 'Kindly circling back on the below. Would you be interested in setting up a time to speak with . . .? This would be a fantastic opportunity to learn about how they are revolutionizing . . .'

Now, I have deliberately chosen some of the worst examples of the way the vast army of public relations professionals try to grab the attention of technology journalists. But PR is a multifaceted industry, with companies employing in-house teams as well as turning to external agencies to get their message across. The latter are often staffed by young people fresh out of university, who sometimes appear to be told by their superiors that quantity matters more than quality: just batter every journalist you can find, no matter how unlikely they are to be interested in your client, until one of them submits and writes something.

At the other end of the spectrum, I know and trust a number of excellent PR people who have a deep understanding of how my organization works, what kind of stories interest our viewers, listeners and readers, and how best to bring them alive. Some of them have even become good friends – after all, many have gone into public relations after a career in journalism, so we have a lot in common.

But I have never bought into the idea they often advance that we are all in this together; that we are basically on the same side. Their job is to paint the tech industry and its products in the best possible light, while ours is to explain this world to our audiences and give some insights into why it is exciting, while retaining a certain critical distance.

And I will admit that, faced with this formidable chorus of hucksters and hype-merchants, we journalists have not always done a great job. Whether it was the Steve Jobs reality-distortion field or Mark

Zuckerberg's philanthropic mission to connect the world, or dozens of start-ups touted as the next big thing, we have sometimes been too slow to pull back the curtain and see the shabby reality behind the technology industry's shiny promises. In the battle between the spinners and the spun, the tech PR army has largely come out on top. But every now and then, the façade has crumbled and the truth has emerged about the failings of a technology company, despite the best efforts of its public relations team. Often that is the result of a brave whistleblower stepping forward.

That was what happened in 2009 when I received an email which, thankfully, I did not delete without reading. It was from an employee of a company called SpinVox. I knew it well – after all, it was a fast-growing UK firm with some radical technology, and I had been so impressed by the service it offered that I had become a customer.

In the days before the term machine learning had become familiar, SpinVox had automated the process of turning voicemails into text. Its website explained that its technology 'captures spoken words and feeds them into a Voice Message Conversion System, known as "D2" (the Brain)'. The system seemed extraordinarily advanced, with the computer making very few mistakes as it turned a garbled voice message into readily understandable text. All very clever and, at a time when voicemail was an important feature of a mobile phone – and before we knew much about how simple it was for unscrupulous journalists to hack one – this was an attractive service. SpinVox was available in seven countries and four languages, earning revenue from individuals and from mobile phone operators wanting to offer customers something hi-tech to differentiate them from their rivals. 'The simplicity is compelling,' chief executive and co-founder Christina Domecq said in 2008 as the firm unveiled a new funding round which, according to a site called Private Equity International, brought the total it had raised to around £200 million. Backers included such blue-chip names as Goldman Sachs and the Carphone Warehouse founder Charles Dunstone, and the new money would allow the business to expand into new languages and territories. I had put the company on television a couple of times and, at a period when new UK tech firms were thin on the ground, SpinVox appeared to me to be just the kind of business we should be celebrating. Then that email arrived.

'Dear Roy', it began, unpromisingly. Then it perked up: 'I think I have a very interesting story for you. Please look at the following links. I am currently employed with SpinVox and provide you with a lot more background.' The links were to a couple of items on the SpinVox website – the funding announcement from the previous year and the company's privacy policy – and several news stories.

One was a suggestion that the firm was paying staff in stock to save on costs. Another concerned the previous track record of the management. But it was a link to an obscure blog about 'what's shaking in the world of voicemail transcription' that caught my eye. There was a post with the title 'SpinVox humans', with some photos of what might be a call centre, and a computer monitor showing what appeared to be a voicemail message about some complex financial transaction. What exactly was going on here?

I called the author of the email. He did not want to say more over the phone, but suggested we meet. So it was that a couple of days later I went to a café near my West London home for one of the more extraordinary encounters of my career in journalism.

My contact, who arrived carrying a laptop, was a member of the security team at SpinVox. Connecting his computer to the café's Wi-Fi, he took me inside the company's system. His first revelation was that an organization which was storing on its servers all kinds of sensitive messages from the voicemails of thousands of customers had appalling security.

He accessed the system using the login and very simple password of a former colleague who had left the company, pointing out how easy it would be for this person to cause mischief. He then took me on a tour of the operation, which soon revealed what appeared to be a devastating truth about the way the voicemail-to-text transcription worked. For the most part, it looked like it was done not by machines but by humans.

He pointed me to a graph showing the percentage of text messages that were processed by what SpinVox referred to in its press releases as its 'ground-breaking Voice Message Conversion System™ (VMCS), which works by combining state-of-the-art speech technologies with a live-learning language process'. This was represented by an orange line running very low along the y axis: it seemed just one message in ten was transcribed automatically.

The vast majority of messages, he explained, were actually listened to and transcribed by people in call centres around the world: in the Philippines, South Africa, Kenya and Pakistan. Then he showed me some of my own messages, with evidence of which call centre had handled them. He pointed me to some posts on Facebook where call-centre employees in Egypt had discussed their work transcribing messages for SpinVox. Later, I managed to reach one of them on the phone, who confirmed that his job had been to read messages – and also that there had been issues with payments, which had led to this particular call centre ending its relationship with SpinVox.

That brought us to another element of the whistleblower's tale, which related to the story he had sent me about staff being asked to take their salary in shares rather than cash. He told me about a recent all-hands meeting where the chief executive and co-founder Christina Domecq had admitted that the entire future of the business depended on the staff taking that option. He even showed me a video of the event. 'This is the tipping point in our redefining of the speech industry,' we watched Domecq saying, and going on to talk about the actions necessary over the next six weeks 'to get through the storm'.

It was obvious when you thought about it. The whole premise of the business was that the transcription process was largely automated, and therefore more cost-effective. So if instead you had to employ thousands of staff in call centres around the world, then the numbers didn't add up. As evidence of how the finances were under strain, the whistleblower showed me emails revealing that SpinVox had been shut out of one of its data centres after failing to pay its bills, just as the Egyptian source had said.

This, then, was a story with three strands. First, one of the UK's most exciting young companies had overhyped its technology. Secondly, by sending messages for call-centre workers around the world to read, it appeared to have broken data protection laws, having guaranteed that none of its data would be processed outside the EU. And finally, it was in financial trouble, with its blue-chip backers almost certainly unaware of just how badly off course the company was heading.

I left the café both very excited about the story and painfully aware of how much work needed to be done before we could go public with it. The next couple of days involved a blizzard of phone calls – with SpinVox's substantial PR team, with my editors and with a BBC lawyer.

The company quickly saw that this story could be a real threat to its existence, and put me in touch with Daniel Doulton, the less colourful of its two co-founders. Doulton, a member of the family behind the Royal Doulton china business – his co-founder Christina Domecq was part of the Spanish drinks dynasty – was quietly spoken and earnest. SpinVox had always said there was some human involvement, he maintained, but the majority of calls were processed by machines. He insisted that no data protection laws were being broken because the message data was merely being processed, not stored, abroad. And yes, like any business it had faced challenges, but it was now profitable.

I was pretty confident that all three statements were inaccurate, having seen the evidence presented by my whistleblower. In the meantime I had also talked to a couple of other insiders. But without anyone willing to go on the record, we would have to proceed carefully. We offered SpinVox the right to reply, and there was talk from their PR team of a television interview with Daniel Doulton or some other executive.

That failed to materialize and, after multiple drafts of the story and many late-night conversations with the BBC lawyer who, while cautious, was determined to help get this story out, we were ready to publish. On a July morning a few days after my meeting with the whistleblower, my report headlined 'The Spinning of SpinVox' went up on the BBC news website. That same morning I appeared on Radio 4's *Today* programme to talk about my story with the presenter, Evan Davis. Unusually, my live exchange with Evan was scripted – the lawyer had insisted it would be too dangerous for me to just extemporize as normal.

I explained what SpinVox was – most of the audience would never have heard of the company – and what it claimed about its technology. Then I went through the headlines of what I had learned. 'I've been told by a company insider that the majority of calls are actually transcribed not by clever machines but by call-centre staff around the world. I've also spoken to a former call-centre worker in Egypt who did some of the work, and seen evidence that my own calls are actually transcribed in this way.'

Evan asked why any of this mattered. I outlined the data protection issues around customer information leaving Europe and then being listened to by call-centre staff. And I explained that the company's finances depended on getting machines, not humans, to do the work. That SpinVox had just asked its staff to take their pay in shares, not cash, for the next two months, showed the strain it was under.

I then reported the company's statement, which said SpinVox complied with all data protection laws and met the highest security standards at home and abroad, with all messages encrypted and anonymized. But I concluded by saying I had repeatedly asked what proportion of messages were dealt with entirely by machines rather than humans, and that the company had refused to tell me, citing commercial confidentiality.

While I was very excited by the story I was realistic enough to know that it was not going to make it beyond the website and this early-morning radio slot. Getting on a television bulletin means clearing a high hurdle, and editors were not going to see this as one of the major stories of the day. Nevertheless, my online article made a big impact, and was picked up by technology news sites around the world. Even the *Wall Street Journal* covered it, with the headline, 'A Voicemail Transcription Scandal in Britain'.

But very rapidly SpinVox, its PR machine and its supporters swung into action, trying to knock the story down. First out of the blocks was a blogpost from the entrepreneur and financier Julie Meyer. I had met Julie years earlier when I interviewed her for my book about the UK's dot.com bubble. She had been one of the founders of the networking group First Tuesday, and had fallen out with her colleagues over the proceeds of the sale of what was effectively an overhyped wine-and-cheese party. Now she seemed determined to fall out with me. 'SpinVox is a turbo-charged, over-the-top success story of which the UK should be enormously proud,' she wrote, saying she was proud to have equity in the firm – it later emerged that she had a negligible stake. She went on to hint that in trying to pull down its chief executive Christina Domecq I was guilty both of misogyny and tall-poppy syndrome: 'It's only the small-minded, insecure or jealous who would pull someone down who is the biggest and best example this country has had for a very long time of how to lead the team, and how to build an incredibly valuable company from a simple, smart idea.'

Then the SpinVox in-house blogger James Whatley, an engaging fellow who went by the handle Whatleydude, published a lengthy rebuttal. He went through my allegations one by one, and tried to dismiss them in a chatty, informal style. On the key question of what proportion of messages were converted into text by machines rather than humans he wrote this:

> Well I'll be honest with you folks, I've been wrestling away with this one most of today. I wish I could tell you, really I could. But this information is so business critical to our operation that we simply cannot share it. I'm not kidding when I say that it would be the equivalent of Coca-Cola publishing their exact recipe up on their own blog.

I wrote another piece, rebutting Whatleydude's rebuttal. I felt a bit sorry for him: insiders from the firm's technology division were telling me that he and the marketing team did not really understand just how poorly the system was performing. A month or so later he moved on from SpinVox.

But by now *PR Week* was reporting that SpinVox had launched 'a major PR offensive in response to potentially damaging claims by the BBC'. The blue-chip financial PR firm Brunswick had been hired to shore up the defences, working alongside the in-house team and a consumer agency. They came up with a brilliant plan. Journalists and bloggers – although not the BBC – were invited to an event at the firm's headquarters in Marlow, where the amazing technology would be demonstrated.

The event began to unravel even before it happened, with one blogger refusing to attend because SpinVox would not allow him to film the demo 'on security grounds'. Those who did show up were shown how, under ideal conditions, the automated system could turn around a message in about four seconds. But most journalists left unimpressed both by the demo and by the answers to their questions to Christina Domecq, when she made a brief appearance. Andrew Orlowski of the *Register* was on particularly acerbic form: 'All but one of the messages – a simple one placed by the SpinVox chief technology officer in a silent room – tripped through to the Tenzing console for manual interpretation. Pretty much in their entirety. So much for call center staff, sorry, agents, only seeing occasional word fragments.'

But as the summer wore on it was the finances of the company rather than its technology that became the focus. The most recent published accounts had shown that in 2007 SpinVox had revenues of just £2 million and made a loss of £36 million. Such figures were not unusual then – or now – in a fast-growing tech start-up. But one figure stood out: the £546,000 salary paid to the chief executive Christina Domecq.

More began to emerge about the track record of Domecq and her co-founder Daniel Doulton. One company they had run in the United States had gone bankrupt, owing more than $2 million, and there was talk of lavish spending at SpinVox. More sources came forward, including an employee of an Irish company that was involved in the 'processing' of the messages. He told me they were having trouble getting paid and said, 'It's only a matter of time before the company folds.' As I was still using the SpinVox service – I wanted to keep an eye on what was happening – I asked him whether I should be worried about my own security.

'They are listening to every message they convert,' he said. 'And if I was to notify anyone of a message all I'd have to do is take note of an ID number for the message when it's converted, and they can rehear it over and over again. Be very wary.'

Then I began to hear reports of an explosive document: an anonymous letter that had been sent to Goldman Sachs and other investors. It apparently consisted of allegations of accounting irregularities, misrepresentation of the state of the company's finances and lurid details of the misuse of company funds for personal expenses. I obviously needed to get hold of this document, and I started to work my sources to see if they could help. Eventually, someone came forward and, in true cloak-and-dagger style, we met for a cup of tea at the hotel at Paddington Station. The source did not hand over the document there and then but, a couple of days later, a brown envelope landed on my doormat at home.

As I skimmed through the document two things immediately became clear. It had been written by someone with intimate knowledge of the company and its finances and, if the picture it painted was accurate, the investors had been taken for a very expensive ride by the management.

The letter appeared to show just how false a picture had been painted of the capabilities of the technology. While investors had been told that 70 per cent of messages were transcribed without human involvement, the true figure was more like 10 per cent – which is what my whistleblower had told me. The firm had also under-reported just how much money it was losing for every message, and it had booked revenues from contracts with mobile phone operators that had yet to be signed.

Meanwhile, and most colourfully, money was flowing out of the cash-strapped business to fund a luxury lifestyle for the management. Two sales executives who had made no sales had been given luxury cars, one of them an Aston Martin. But that was just an appetiser compared to the alleged spending on the chief executive Christina Domecq, including a chauffeur-driven BMW 7 Series, and a £100,000 Mercedes for her own use. The letter also appeared to show a racing yacht charged to the company – a mere €457,700 – although this was supposedly to be used to raise the profile of a charity she had founded.

But the highlight was that SpinVox had apparently paid for Ms Domecq's wedding on a private island, including the costs of having guests flown in from around the world. In all, the letter said, she was taking more than £1 million a year out of a business that was struggling to pay either its staff or its suppliers.

What a story. Except that, once I had spoken to the lawyers and my editor, it became clear there was nothing we could publish. We had just one source – the anonymous letter writer – and that was not enough, as we could not prove its contents. I set about contacting former members of the finance team and the investors to try to verify some of the contents of the letter. But nobody wanted to go on the record. It became apparent that the investors, embarrassed by their failure to keep an eye on what was happening with their money, just wanted to move on.

A few months later SpinVox was swallowed up by Nuance, an American firm with a much longer track record in voice-to-text technology, for $102 million – about £64 million at that time. That sounded like quite a decent price for an ailing business, and one might imagine the firm's backers would have been quite pleased with themselves.

But a few weeks later the truth emerged. Just about all of that £64 million had gone to pay off the emergency loans that had kept the company afloat during the crisis in the summer. The investors, from Goldman Sachs and Charles Dunstone to the dozens of staff who had taken shares in lieu of payment, got just £600. No, not each. That was spread between all of them.

As I wrote at the time, it was just about the biggest destruction of shareholder value I had seen since the dot.com bubble, after which many shares were fit only to paper the bathroom wall.

Christina Domecq disappeared, and resurfaced a few years later in New Zealand, where she started a number of new businesses. I googled her recently, and the most recent news was a story headlined 'Domecq opts for bankruptcy as Aussie investors close in.'

And as for that anonymous letter to investors? Following the take-over by Nuance a filing to America's SEC (Securities and Exchange Commission) revealed that Domecq had agreed to pay back £125,000 after an investigation into her expenses. A couple of years later the letter was published in full by a London tech scandal sheet. By then, though, the whole affair had faded from view and the London tech scene had moved on to the next big shiny thing.

I have spent some time on the SpinVox affair, partly because it was a story that I was so heavily involved in and enjoyed hugely, but also because it seemed to capture some of the most unattractive aspects of the smartphone era: a tendency for technology businesses to oversell their products, and an overweening arrogance among entrepreneurs who believed their own hype, supported by their legions of PR apparatchiks and by short-sighted investors.

There were plenty more examples of tech firms and products that failed to live up to the hype – sometimes because of deliberate deception, but often because both the spinners and the spun, the PRs and the journalists, just got over-excited about products that were not ready for mainstream adoption – or might never be.

Take Google Glass, for instance. This experimental headset, which allowed you to livestream what you were doing, take pictures and videos with a voice command, and get news and social media updates in a tiny screen in front of your eye, was first shown off at Google's annual I/O (Input/Output) conference in 2012. I thought it looked amazing, and a year later managed to persuade the BBC to send me and a film crew to California to shoot a story about it. My interest grew ever greater and, when it became available in limited numbers for software developers to buy in 2014 for £1,500, I made an impassioned case to the BBC technology division that we should get one for me to test on a long-term basis. I was convinced that this could be the most exciting, groundbreaking new product since the iPhone, so I needed to assess it.

For three months, I travelled around with this pair of space-age spectacles, taking pictures, making short films, and asking people what they thought of what I was wearing. I wore them at a football match, while jogging with my dog, even while having a dental examination. Many laughed, including my family and colleagues; some were intrigued, and a few found the idea of the spy in my eye creepy rather than cool.

The problem was, I eventually realized, that Google Glass was not creepy, not cool – just faintly ridiculous. A few months after I stopped using it, Google announced that it was halting sales, although development would continue in a more low-key way. But the headset never made a return, one of a number of failures from the mighty search engine company, which has struggled when it comes to building hardware that people might want to pay for. Here was a lesson about the gap between hype and reality: wealthy companies that had achieved great breakthroughs in one area could then deploy vast marketing budgets to promote their next big idea, but all too often they were over-confident in their own judgement of what consumers wanted from technology.

A case in point is the wave of investment and hype in both virtual reality and augmented reality, where virtual objects are overlaid on the real world. VR, which had failed in the 1990s because it made users feel seasick, was supposedly coming back in a big way, with upstart companies like Oculus Rift, swiftly snapped up by Facebook, leading the charge.

Billions were poured into virtual-reality games, and then, when gamers failed to show sufficient interest, the focus switched to VR's use in business, education and healthcare. I was shown a variety of potential uses: training an engineer how to assemble a satellite dish in remote terrain without them needing to actually travel there. Or helping someone terrified of getting into lifts to overcome their phobia.

After a couple of years, the press releases about virtual reality were replaced by those touting augmented reality – a far more 'relatable' technology, apparently. Apple was getting into the technology in a big way; an American start-up company called Magic Leap produced a demo that so enthralled investors, they poured $3.5 billion into it; a London business called Blippar achieved a $1 billion valuation as it showed off tech that would make a Spotify track play when you pointed a smartphone camera at a can of Coke.

But by 2020, Apple still had not showed off the magic augmented-reality glasses 'everyone' knew they were working on, Blippar had collapsed, and Magic Leap appeared to have leaped off a cliff, undone, in the words of a Bloomberg headline, by profligate spending and its own hype.

Sometimes it was not just the tech but the people selling it that were massively oversold. In 2012 I began to receive regular emails from a PR agency representing Dan Wagner, chief executive of a company called Powa Technologies.

Powa was apparently set to revolutionize the way we shopped, with a variety of mobile payment devices and services, including the PowaTag, 'which enables consumers to purchase goods by tagging a code on any surface or audio from advertisements or radio.'

It seemed I really needed to meet Dan, whose 'whole life has been built on tech innovation' and 'who has created dynamic e-commerce technology solutions for high street names such as Tesco, Superdrug, Laura Ashley and Heal's'. Dan was not just a brilliant innovator: he was also a seasoned commentator, available for interviews on news from the retail industry. 'This will be a wake-up call for many retailers that are sleep-walking into turmoil,' hollered Dan Wagner, in just one of his many piercing insights supplied by the PR agency.

Then there was exciting news from Powa, 'the UK e-commerce/ m-commerce leader' of a record $76 million investment from a

US equity firm, creating almost 500 jobs. And, wow, 'Dan Wagner, the CEO of Powa Technologies, has had the backing of the Prime Minister on this deal.' It was true, David Cameron had provided a statement: 'E-commerce is vital to our economic success,' he had said. 'That is why this expansion of Powa is such good news – helping British Business increase trade both at home and abroad.'

Still I did not bite, and the tone of the PR emails grew increasingly forlorn: 'I have been reaching out to you about Powa Technologies for some time now and I have some news that might actually interest you.'

In 2014, Powa paid $75 million to acquire a Hong Kong mobile payments start-up, and Dan Wagner proclaimed that his business now had a valuation of $2.6 billion. 'This deal reinforces the perception that PowaTag is the emerging leader, if not the dominant provider, of mobile payment solutions worldwide.'

By now, Powa was obviously one of the UK's most important young technology companies. Its activities were being covered widely, and its chief executive Dan Wagner was being invited onto Sky and, yes, even onto the BBC, to give his views on all manner of tech and retail stories.

But not by me. Because I had a long memory, and knew a little bit about Mr Wagner's extraordinary career.

Back in the 1980s he had started MAID, one of the first online information platforms, and had become, so he claimed, the youngest chief executive of a UK-listed company. He had attracted attention by wearing a Donald Duck waistcoat during the share sale – an early sign of a penchant for showmanship that would become a feature of his career. The *Sunday Times* journalist Andrew Davidson later wrote of how desperate the young Wagner had been for publicity. 'He'd ring, he'd drive round to my office. He was charming but incorrigible, like one of those kids who is told that everything they do is wonderful, and becomes completely insensitive to how others feel or perceive them.'

In the late 1990s MAID was rebranded as Dialog, but as the dot. com bubble burst its share price plunged 95 per cent, and it was rechristened 'Dial a dog' by city analysts. Later, Wagner had moved on to a series of other businesses, before setting up Powa, but his career had been marked by a tendency to make promises about big deals and market dominance which had then failed to materialize. Hence my scepticism, which was only fuelled by the constant stream of breathless press releases from the small PR agency he had hired.

Late in 2015, however, it appeared that Powa had done just the kind of groundbreaking deal that Dan Wagner had long promised. 'A British start-up just scooped Apple in China with an "800lb gorilla" of a deal,' was the excited headline on a *Business Insider* story. Powa's PR firm also approached the BBC with the story that the company had done a deal in China that would see PowaTag gain access to the 1.3 billion customers of China UnionPay, the country's leading force in payments, and open up a new era of mobile commerce. Dan Wagner spoke to a colleague on the BBC's online team. 'Why did China UnionPay decide to partner with a little British technology company? We've trumped Apple Pay and the rest of the world here,' he boasted.

I urged caution, thinking it all sounded like typical Wagner braggadocio, and the next day the story changed. No, it was not an exclusive deal, and Apple had not been trumped: its payment system was arriving in China and was likely to prove more popular than the obscure PowaTag. The PR agency rang my colleague and asked him to remove the quote from the story because Dan Wagner was now embarrassed by it. Naturally, he refused.

Still, with at least some kind of deal in China, surely Powa, which of course had that $2.6 billion valuation, would be going public soon? Wagner told US business news TV channel CNBC it was 'definitely on our radar', and could be possible in 2016, but he was giving 'no commitments'.

Which was fortunate, really, because just a couple of months later the company went spectacularly bust. Its major backer, the American private equity firm Wellington Management – the one whose backing had generated that extraordinary $2.6 billion valuation figure – called in the administrators as it became clear that the money had run out.

Some weeks earlier, I had been told by a couple of insiders that all was not well, and staff were not being paid. Now, an army of whistleblowers came forward, with testimony of just how false a picture the company had painted of its technology and finances, and they had documents to prove it.

That China deal? The team that negotiated it had been horrified by the way it was portrayed. They had told Mr Wagner not to oversell the deal, but he had gone off script. 'He just shot his mouth off,' one person told me. 'The Chinese were furious – they don't like that kind of boasting.' And the supposed partner China UnionPay had sent a 'cease and desist' letter ordering Powa to shut up. 'As a matter of fact', said the letter, 'our company has not yet established any business relationship with your company.'

And while Wagner had bragged of lucrative deals for top brands like L'Oréal and Carrefour to use the PowaTag, they had not signed contracts either: merely letters of intent which did not commit them to anything. Then there were tales of lavish spending: huge salaries for the top executives, two floors of the Heron Tower in London and prime office locations in Hong Kong and New York, and dinners and parties which appeared a throwback to the excesses of the 1980s. Several employees described one Christmas bash in Mayfair at which strippers were hired to perform, to the discomfort of many present.

But even as the sky darkened, the staff waited to be paid, and an internal document warned that the company was in danger of trading while insolvent, Dan Wagner remained chipper. In January, he sent an email to all staff with the subject line, 'Long live the legacy of David Bowie.' It was the day after the death of the rock legend had been announced, and the email featured a photo of their chief executive dressed as Ziggy Stardust in full make-up, with the caption: 'I don't do tributes in half measures!'

It is safe to say the employees were not impressed. As one put it to me, 'While the company was going under, he's fooling around in a photography studio pretending to be Ziggy Stardust. The guy is a narcissistic idiot.'

When I wrote a lengthy article about the collapse of Powa it was headlined, 'The start-up that fell to earth', and the photo of Dan Wagner as Ziggy Stardust featured prominently. He, unsurprisingly, was not happy, about either the article or the photo, and over the months that followed he contacted the BBC repeatedly offering to tell his side of the story. But there was one condition. I must not be involved in any way whatsoever. Nothing came of it, and the irrepressible entrepreneur was soon starting a new business, which appeared to be offering very similar technology to the PowaTag.

Once again a colourful personality, a lack of curiosity from eager investors and the short memories of some journalists had combined to create a picture of groundbreaking technology which bore little resemblance to reality. And there is no reason to believe this kind of story will not be repeated in the coming years.

Some two and a half years later a letter arrived at the BBC from Dan Wagner's lawyers. It stated that the copyright in the Ziggy Stardust photo belonged to their client, and would we please remove it from the article on the website. The BBC's lawyers told us that we did not have a watertight defence on this, so it would be wiser to comply. Several other news organizations apparently received similar letters, and the photo disappeared from view.

The UK had its share of overpraised, oversold companies whose technology failed to live up to the image their PR teams successfully marketed to hard-pressed journalists, but as ever there were bigger and better examples in the United States. Theranos promised a revolutionary blood test from a prick of the finger, and its founder Elizabeth Holmes was touted by *Fortune* magazine as the next Steve Jobs – until a brilliant investigative journalist at the *Wall Street Journal* laid bare a tale of failed technology and blindsided investors.

Meanwhile WeWork, a business leasing funky office space to start-ups, somehow managed to convince the world and its big backer SoftBank that it was a technology growth company worth as much as $47 billion. A breathless analyst's report described how WeWork achieved maximum efficiency in its buildings through its use of machine learning, with its researchers creating a 'neural net' that collected information on layouts and meeting-room usage.

Only when the company had to publish more details of its finances as it prepared for an IPO did the familiar story of lavish spending, overhyped or non-existent technology and the fantastical pretensions of its founder – Adam Neumann's ambition for WeWork was to 'elevate the world's consciousness' – become clear, bringing everything crashing down. The IPO never happened, and what was just another property business set about the struggle to survive the coronavirus pandemic.

In the smartphone era, the public might feel justifiably aggrieved by the picture they receive of technology. One minute they are told that Silicon Valley rock stars are inventing the future, with gadgets that will transform their lives for the better. The next, they learn that the tech titans are evil manipulators, stealing your data and hyping all kinds of products that are of little value and may cause you harm.

So who is to blame for this: the spinners, the businesses that employ them, or the journalists who swallow their stories? I convened a couple of my friends in PR to discuss this. Let's not use their real names – they hope to continue their long and successful careers which have seen them represent major American and European technology companies both for external agencies and in-house. So I will call them Jane and Patrick.

Jane sympathized with me about the tidal wave of nonsense that arrives in my inbox. 'I really feel journalists are just bombarded with crap, basically.' But she pinned the blame not on the agencies but on their clients. Too many tech company bosses just didn't understand the media – 'There's a quite staggering level of media illiteracy.' As a veteran of the industry, she now had the confidence to push back against 'executives who are trying to get me and my team to come to people like you with what I would say are weak or bad stories.'

Patrick, who started off as a newspaper journalist, felt too many young fresh-faced PR people at agencies were 'just not experienced enough or investing the time to get up to speed before they actually pick up the phone to journalists.' Mind you, he also thought that 20 years ago there was a smaller, more specialist band of reporters – 'proper hardcore tech journalists' – who really knew their stuff and could not have the wool pulled over their eyes.

Both look on with a mixture of admiration and horror at the Apple PR operation, and its iron discipline at getting its message across. 'The media have partly created that beast,' said Patrick, 'and actually have given them an easy ride.' I remarked just what a challenge it is to get anything out of Apple. I once spent months negotiating to get an interview with the chief executive, Tim Cook, at a major product launch. While we had never had an interview with Steve Jobs' successor, the signs were hopeful. But a couple of weeks before the event I was called in to Apple's London office to be told that an exclusive had been granted to the anchor of one of the American nightly news programmes.

To my horror, I watched his folksy piece begin with him actually hugging Tim Cook as he came off stage after unveiling the new product. Not a sequence I could ever imagine in a British television news piece.

Jane, who spent much of her career at another giant American tech firm, acknowledged that there is a cultural difference between US and British journalists, which makes it hard for her to persuade executives to engage with the likes of me. 'They see you guys as cynical, negative, out to embarrass or trip people up. And they don't necessarily see that the benefit of engaging is worth the potential cost of engaging.'

Jane and Patrick both understood why there had been a 'techlash': a revolt against the tech companies, and their belief that they were ushering in a new borderless utopia where local laws were of little relevance. 'There was a reckoning needed,' said Jane. 'There's a dreadful arrogance in this industry.'

Let's leave the last word to the whistleblower who alerted me to what was happening inside SpinVox. In 2020, I got back in touch with him, and found that he was still working as a software engineer, but was now based abroad. We chatted somewhat nostalgically about our 'Deep Throat' encounter in that café in Ealing more than a decade earlier. He explained what had made him take the big step of contacting me. 'I just got sick of the lies,' he said. 'I couldn't actually do my job. It was just the frustration, the disconnect between what I was hearing and what I was seeing.'

He said he had been a naive young technologist when we met, shocked by what was going on at SpinVox. But he had learned over the years to be a lot more sceptical. 'When I read a news article or a press release and stuff like that, I ask myself, which is real technology and how much is promise?' And he said artificial intelligence, the field in which SpinVox had claimed to be making huge advances, was the classic example. 'Half the AI companies are over-promising and under-delivering, because the technology isn't mature.' We talked about the mismatch between the long-term research that is behind every advance in technology, and the short-term need for publicity – and cash from investors – that drives the overblown claims and hysterical press releases.

After saying goodbye, I reflected that the technology SpinVox had been touting, machine learning, which enabled the efficient conversion of voice into text, had since come a long way. I had just recorded my conversation with the whistleblower using a transcription app which provided a reasonably accurate account of his words. AI was making some progress, even if it did not match up to the PR promises. But as for another revolutionary technology which, according to its boosters, was going to be even bigger than the internet, I was increasingly sceptical that it would ever deliver.

10

Crypto Craziness

April 2016, and in the offices of a PR agency in London's Soho, I waited anxiously with my producer for a meeting that was about to deliver the biggest scoop of my career as a technology journalist. In the next few minutes, the mysterious figure behind a revolution that looked set to transform the way the world's financial system worked would be sitting in front of me proving his identity. Or so I had been promised.

Six weeks earlier I had been contacted by an executive from the Outside Organization, which was a major player in the music industry, having represented everyone from David Bowie to the Spice Girls. Slightly bizarre, then, that the PR agent should be promising to give me a huge technology story, but I was intrigued and agreed to meet. A few days later, I was informed that I was going to be one of just three journalists to meet Satoshi Nakamoto. Well, I reflected: if that was true, this was a very juicy story indeed.

In 2009, a paper was published online with the title, 'Bitcoin: A Peer-to-Peer Electronic Cash System'. It set out, over nine pages, with plenty of technical detail and a scattering of equations, a proposal for an electronic cash system. What was revolutionary about it was that it was decentralized: no bank or government would control this currency, which would be created by a computing process and governed by cryptography, rather than by any mechanism of trust between institutions and individuals.

The author of the paper was Satoshi Nakamoto, and, in the seven years since its publication, his idea had taken off – or at least had won over an army of disciples. Some of them were technologists enthused by the elegance of the concept; some were libertarians who loved the idea of upending the global financial system; many were speculators or individuals eager to find ways of moving money without the oversight of regulators or law enforcement agencies.

Online sellers of illicit goods, from drugs to guns, quickly adopted this cryptocurrency as their payment method of choice, confident it was untraceable. That confidence took a hit when the FBI shut down the Silk Road marketplace, seizing 26,000 Bitcoin and arresting its swashbuckling owner Dread Pirate Roberts – or, more prosaically, Ross William Ulbricht.

Bitcoin, as measured by its value against the dollar, had already been through a number of booms and busts, spiking up to $31 in 2011, before collapsing to $2, then climbing above $1,000 at Christmas 2013, before halving in value again. I had produced my first stories on the virtual currency in 2013, acquiring some from a Bitcoin cash machine and buying a pizza with it for Radio 4's *PM* programme. It was a cumbersome process, which saw me acquire one small Papa John's pizza with anchovies, black olives and mushrooms for 0.3249 Bitcoin – about £30 then, but worth about £10,000 when the currency surged above $50,000 in early 2021. That experience, and other attempts to buy things at the few cafés and shops accepting the currency, had convinced me that Bitcoin was not yet much use, except as a means of speculation.

But interest in Bitcoin was accelerating, with an army of consultancies and analysts still predicting that cryptocurrencies and their underlying technology, blockchain, were going to be the next big thing – perhaps even more transformative than the internet.

Meanwhile, the mystery about the identity of its creator deepened. In the early days Satoshi Nakamoto had communicated with a few enthusiasts helping to build out his vision for Bitcoin, and had made the occasional public pronouncement. But then he had faded from view. As journalists tried to identify him there were a number of theories. Was he Japanese, or was the name a diversion, behind which hid an American? Many thought there was a group of people, probably in the United States rather than Japan, who had come together behind the Nakamoto brand to publish the paper and create the currency. There was even a discussion about whether Nakamoto was in fact British, after textual analysis revealed his skilled use of apostrophes and the Oxford comma.

Then in 2014 it seemed that *Newsweek* had come up trumps. A story headlined 'The Face Behind Bitcoin' revealed that Dorian Nakamoto, a 64-year-old Japanese-American retired physicist and model train collector living in California, was Satoshi Nakamoto, hiding in plain sight. The story quickly fell apart, however, with Mr Nakamoto insisting that a quote he had given to the *Newsweek* journalist – 'I am no longer involved in that and I cannot discuss it' – had been misunderstood, referring to his career in engineering rather than being an admission of past involvement in the currency.

But speculation about the identity of Satoshi became ever more feverish, and in 2016 a lot of it centred on an Australian computer scientist and businessman. So when a door opened in those Soho offices that April morning and I was ushered in, I was not entirely surprised to find Craig Wright sitting in front of me.

A few months earlier, two tech publications, *Wired* and *Gizmodo*, had suggested Wright – or Dr Wright, as he styled himself, claiming to have doctorates in theology and computer science – was Satoshi. But that unleashed a maelstrom of claim and counterclaim in the noisily argumentative Bitcoin community, with many convinced that this was another false trail.

A few hours after the article was published, the Australian police raided Wright's home in New South Wales, allegedly as part of a tax investigation. Then, a few days later, *Wired* revealed that its original investigation had been launched after it had received a collection of emails and other documents from a mysterious source close to Craig Wright, backing up the claim that he was the Bitcoin inventor. Having looked more closely at the evidence, the magazine now suspected it had been the target of an elaborate hoax.

Now, though, in 2016, the BBC, along with the *Economist* and *GQ* magazine, were to be given conclusive proof that Craig Wright was indeed the genius who had written that paper back in 2009, and gone on to shape the currency of the future. We were told that he would use cryptographic keys from the early days of Bitcoin known to have been associated with Satoshi to sign a document.

When I walked into the conference room there were four people sitting around a table, and I was not sure at first which one was Wright, until I realized that the man staring intently at a laptop, failing to greet us or even acknowledge our presence, must be him.

At first it promised to be a deeply uncomfortable encounter. He made it clear that he did not really want to be there, and suggested that others had put pressure on him to come out of the shadows. It later emerged that he was linked to a web of companies involved in Bitcoin activities financed by a Canadian casino billionaire, Calvin Ayre. Craig Wright and the host of patent applications he seemed to post on an almost daily basis were at the heart of this business, and later Calvin Ayre's Coingeek cryptocurrency blog would vigorously promote a series of libel cases against anyone who suggested his protégé was not Satoshi.

Gradually Wright warmed up, and eventually he performed the demonstration that had been promised to show he did have access to Satoshi's cryptographic keys. The process was pretty much incomprehensible to anyone unfamiliar with the inner workings of cryptocurrencies, but in the room was Jon Matonis, a senior figure in the Bitcoin world, who vouched for the claims about what we had seen. We were also put in touch with Gavin Andresen, chief scientist of the Bitcoin Foundation, who had been given a similar demonstration and seemed convinced.

Once he'd relaxed, Wright seemed content to answer our questions. He produced a series of documents to prove he had the academic credentials his denigrators said were imaginary, dismissed the Australian tax investigation as the result of a misunderstanding about the nature of Bitcoin, and said the name Nakamoto came from a seventeenth-century libertarian philosopher. The origin of 'Satoshi', however, was something he would keep to himself.

By now the founder of Bitcoin should have been as rich as Croesus, but he wouldn't reveal how many coins he owned, insisting that although he lived in a big house in London and drove a fast car he was not particularly motivated by money.

As far as our story was concerned, we now needed to seal the deal with a second meeting, where we would interview him on camera and get him saying 'I am Satoshi.' But when we returned to the PR agency a few days later his mood had darkened. At first it seemed he would not do an interview at all, and his PR executive kept shuttling back and forth to the conference room looking increasingly stressed. Then, when we did get through the door, it was immediately clear that Wright hated the whole process of being filmed, refusing to move from behind his laptop to a more spacious room where the shot would have been much better.

Then a painful negotiation ensued, with him insisting that he would give an answer to just one question: why he had decided to go public after all these years. Once we started filming he let his guard down a little, but mainly because he wanted to express his anger at what he saw as being forced into the public eye. 'I don't want money. I don't want fame. I don't want adoration. I just want to be left alone!' he said, with some venom. He accused journalists of threatening to make up stories about him if he did not co-operate, and said lies had been told which would affect his family and his staff. And getting him to say he was Satoshi proved an agonizing business. Here is how the conversation went as he prepared to sign a message with the public cryptographic key of Satoshi:

> *Me*: So you're going to show me that Satoshi Nakamoto is you.
> *Craig Wright*: Yes. Some people will believe, some people won't.
>   And to tell you the truth, I don't really care.
> *Me*: But you can say, hand on heart to me, 'I am Satoshi Nakamoto'?
> *Craig Wright*: I was the main part of it. Other people helped me.

That was the best we were going to get. The interview ended with him saying that this was the only time he would ever do this. 'I will never, *ever*, be on a camera ever again. For any TV station, or any media.' So at least we really did have a world television exclusive.

We agreed that we would wait to broadcast the interview until the morning a few days later when he published his public declaration about being Satoshi, accompanied by documentary proof. This came in the form of a blogpost, which started by quoting Schopenhauer:

All truth passes through three stages.
First, it is ridiculed.
Second, it is violently opposed.
Third, it is accepted as being self-evident.

The somewhat self-important Dr Wright went on to compare himself with Jean-Paul Sartre, who turned down the pre-eminent literary prize because he did not want to be known for ever as Jean-Paul Sartre, Nobel Prizewinner, just as Dr Wright did not want to be known as Craig 'Satoshi' Wright. It was the text of Sartre's speech declining the Nobel which he signed and encrypted with the private key associated with Satoshi and an early block of newly minted Bitcoins.

The post was published early on 2 May. A few hours later, the interview with Wright had been broadcast, my lengthy article was published on the BBC website, and I talked about the story on Radio 4's *Today* programme. A great scoop, then? Well, not quite.

Very quickly things began to fall apart. That very day leading lights from the Bitcoin community were gathering in New York for a conference called Consensus – and the only topic of conversation was the unmasking of Satoshi. As various cryptography wizards began to delve into Craig Wright's 'proof', doubts quickly grew. Gavin Andresen, the most credible witness to the demo in London, said he still believed that the Australian was the real deal but, as he was chased around the conference by camera crews, he appeared increasingly anxious.

Within hours, evidence emerged from the crypto experts that Wright could have simply copied an earlier transaction in which Satoshi's private key had been used: he definitely had not proved he had access to that key, they said. By now, I was in a difficult position. While we had not said Craig Wright was Satoshi, merely that he had identified himself as the father of Bitcoin, we were not looking too clever – 'gullible', was how a snarky piece in the *Financial Times* put it.

We asked for more evidence, and by the next day Craig Wright and his spin machine were promising they would go further, and provide 'extraordinary proof' of his claims. An email arrived: 'In the coming days Dr Wright will provide further evidence as to him being Satoshi and the creator of Bitcoin by moving a coin from an early block.'

Well, that sounded good – those early blocks of Bitcoin had lain dormant ever since they had been created. Whoever owned the private key to the blocks was now sitting on an enormous fortune, and spending a tiny bit of it would be convincing proof of his identity.

After a bit of to-ing and fro-ing a scheme was arranged whereby I, Jon Matonis and Gavin Andresen – who by now appeared to be regretting ever having got involved – would send a tiny sum to the Bitcoin address used in the first ever transaction. Then Craig Wright would send it back, in what would be the first outgoing transaction from the block since its creation in January 2009.

I sent my contribution – 0.017 BTC, or about £5 at that time – and then we positioned a camera in front of the web page showing the ledger address where my sum was recorded, along with those from Matonis and Andresen, with a green arrow indicating it was money coming in. What we were waiting for was a red arrow showing Bitcoin coming out.

We waited. And waited. Hours passed, and nothing happened. Then I got a call from the PR agency to say the operation was 'on hold', with no further explanation as to what was happening. The following day Craig Wright published another blogpost on his website, from which all previous posts had been removed. This time, the message was brief and stark:

> *I'm Sorry*
> *I believed that I could do this. I believed that I could put the years of anonymity and hiding behind me. But, as the events of this week unfolded and I prepared to publish the proof of access to the earliest keys, I broke. I do not have the courage. I cannot.*

When the rumors began, my qualifications and character were attacked. When those allegations were proven false, new allegations have already begun. I know now that I am not strong enough for this.

I know that this weakness will cause great damage to those that have supported me, and particularly to Jon Matonis and Gavin Andresen. I can only hope that their honour and credibility is not irreparably tainted by my actions. They were not deceived, but I know that the world will never believe that now. I can only say I'm sorry.

And goodbye.

There was something deeply disturbing about the finality of the last two words, and that was compounded when I took a phone call from someone close to Craig Wright, indicating that he had suffered a depressive episode and might have tried to harm himself. My BBC superiors and I were worried about this, and after one brief blogpost explaining what had happened – without mentioning the phone call – I stepped away from the story.

The whole experience was deeply bruising, and left me cynical about anything surrounding Bitcoin, other cryptocurrencies and the underlying technology blockchain. Spending time with people immersed in this world continued to heighten my suspicions that it bore a close resemblance to the music business as described by Hunter S. Thompson: 'a cruel and shallow money trench, a long plastic hallway where thieves and pimps run free, and good men die like dogs. There's also a negative side.'

As the value of Bitcoin surged upwards towards the $20,000 mark and then fell back again, it continued to be a source of stories. These tended to be about people who had either become hugely wealthy in a big hurry, or had lost a fortune due to fraud or by mislaying the keys to their stash. There was little evidence that Bitcoin was upending the traditional finance system, or becoming a means of exchange or a store of value rather than just a profoundly volatile speculative asset, although it did attract a colourful cast of characters.

Baroness Michelle Mone, the former lingerie entrepreneur who was made a life peer by David Cameron, came up with a scheme to build a Dubai property development, which would be priced and sold in Bitcoin. Why? Apparently it was a chance for those Bitcoin holders who had seen the value of their investment in the cryptocurrency soar to crystallize their profits and put them into less volatile bricks and mortar.

How daring, then, of Baroness Mone and her business and life partner Doug Barrowman to take on the risk of owning all those Bitcoins! Except: they wouldn't. It turned out that the buyers would have to convert their Bitcoin into dollars when they completed their purchase and, although the apartments were 'priced' in Bitcoin, that price would be adjusted in line with the currency's dollar exchange rate. The scheme did attract some investors, and was scheduled for completion in 2019, but by May 2020 it was still a half-finished building site in the middle of a dusty stretch of wasteland. This exciting project had been put on hold the previous year.

But back in 2017 much of the cryptocurrency excitement had moved from Bitcoin to a new phenomenon known as Initial Coin Offerings or ICOs. These combined two revolutionary ideas: one, that the blockchain, the technology underpinning cryptocurrencies, was going to disrupt just about any industry you could imagine; and, two, that creating new currencies for projects using that technology was the road to riches. All you had to do was come up with an idea – say, dentistry on the blockchain – and create a cryptocurrency called Dentacoin to fund it. The idea that a technology start-up would first raise seed capital, then go through several venture capital rounds, before arriving on the stock market via an Initial Public Offering or IPO, was now terribly old hat. An ICO would create magical money from nothing in a matter of months.

Whether you thought this was a great idea depended on how much you bought into the technology of the blockchain: a database stored simultaneously on thousands of computers around the world, with each transaction or piece of data verified by a code (a 'hash') and unchangeable. To true believers, this was as revolutionary as the internet – perhaps more so – because they said it meant trust could be built into a system via cryptography without the need for central control. To sceptics, it was just another database, albeit one with a cult following, where if you put rubbish in, you got rubbish out.

In 2017 there were over 400 successful ICOs, raising an average of nearly $13 million dollars for their promoters, with backers seeing a return of 12.8 times their initial dollar investment, if you looked at the soaring value of the coins they had received. It was a new tulip mania: investors did not really care much about the blockchain projects, or even understand them – they just saw that the value of coins could only go one way.

At least, that was how it seemed when we visited an ICO fair held at a London hotel in early 2018. We were there to start work on a radio documentary about ICOs called *Magical Money*, and wanted to identify a couple of companies whose fortunes we could follow. We wandered round hearing pitches from eager young entrepreneurs who wanted to put radiology or artworks or fine wine on the blockchain, the air thick with jargon about distributed apps, smart contracts and decentralization.

Eventually we settled on two businesses which might at least prove comprehensible to our listeners: BitCar and Viola. BitCar was hoping to raise $25 million for what its founder Gov van Ek, who had already made money from a previous ICO, described as a decentralized platform giving investors a fractional interest in high-end exotic cars.

Come again?

It turned out that BitCar planned to buy a number of McLarens and Ferraris, which the ICO investors would never see – but the tokens they would be given would rise in value along with the cars.

Viola was an even more exotic idea – 'Love on the blockchain', as its Singapore-based founder Violet Lim described it. She was aiming to raise $17 million for a dating agency whose currency would prove valuable to investors in all sorts of ways. 'You can use it to get curated matches, to buy flowers, to book restaurants or even get dating and relationship advice.' I didn't understand why anyone needed a token to buy flowers, or why the dating service needed to be on the blockchain. Ah, explained Viola: it was all about trust – something sadly lacking in the world of dating, but which could be delivered by the distributed-ledger technology. By entering people's details on an immutable blockchain, Viola would be able to deal with 'love scammers' who hide their true identity.

It all seemed extremely far-fetched but, then again, thousands of investors had believed similar stories about the magical properties of the blockchain and been rewarded with spectacular returns in 2017.

It turned out, however, that we had arrived on the ICO scene just as the bubble burst. Perhaps it was because investors had woken up to the fact that the 400 or so success stories of the previous year had been outnumbered by those that had already failed or were in the process of failing. Moreover, this whole decentralized alternative finance industry prided itself on being unregulated and, surprise, surprise, it was turning out to be a fraudster's playground.

The people behind BitCar and Viola appeared sincere in their belief that they had discovered an ingenious way of funding projects that could use the blockchain to deliver services that would help people find love or invest in luxury cars. But when we checked back in with them a couple of months later, a few cracks had appeared in the confident façade they'd presented. BitCar had been aiming to raise $25 million but had only managed $9 million. 'We're not disappointed with that,' insisted the founder, Gov van Ek. 'It's more than enough to get our platform and our vision going.' He accepted that a lot of people were losing faith in the cryptocurrency market but – like everyone else on the ICO scene at that time – he was confident his project would be one of the survivors.

As for dating-on-the-blockchain ICO Viola, it had been even more unfortunate. The public sale of its coins had started on the day in March that Google announced it was banning cryptocurrency and ICO adverts. That, according to Violet Lim, led to 'a very bad first day followed by a very bad first week'. They had decided to 'pause' the sale and monitor market conditions to see when would be a good time to restart.

But market conditions did not improve. In fact, by 2019 the whole concept of an ICO seemed destined to be a tiny footnote in financial history. Viola and BitCar had both released tokens, but they were virtually worthless.

It is unclear what happened to the whole idea of dating on the blockchain. The last time I looked at the Viola website it still linked to an app which talked of harnessing artificial intelligence and blockchain technology to develop 'a lifelong relationship advisor' who would give free advice to singles and couples. But the app had not been updated for a year and had no reviews, so it felt as though the lovelorn might have a lifelong wait for help from Viola.

As for fractional exotic car ownership, soon BitCar was telling its supporters in a blogpost that the dream was over and the platform was closing, despite the 'incredible technical achievements' of the team. 'Unfortunately, BitCar received minimal recognition for the accomplishments due to the very poor sentiment in crypto,' it said. One car, a Ferrari 599 GTO, had been acquired but, rest assured, it was stored safely in immaculate condition awaiting developments rather than being driven around by the founders. The collapse of the business was 'beyond disappointing', and had happened 'despite us having numerous PR agencies engaged and involved in the marketing.'

Given the extent of the disaster that befell the ICO scene – and the increasing evidence that the blockchain was not quite as revolutionary a technology as it had been painted – you might have thought those numerous PR agencies and the whole cryptocurrency marketing industry would have gone quiet for a while.

Not a bit. My inbox continued to fill up with breathless press releases touting blockchain stories – 'Blockchain for Movie Distribution' or 'Blockchain will make online gambling as safe as Las Vegas.' Then there were forecasts that various cryptocurrencies were poised to 'go to the Moon', as the enthusiasts put it, the Moon being a destination where crypto dudes got to drive 'Lambos', or Lamborghinis. Increasingly, I saw the words blockchain or crypto in an email as a cue for instant deletion.

But one March day in 2019 a message arrived that was so startling that I had to read it twice to make sure I had understood it. It was from a PR agency representing a company called Carlauren, which apparently ran care homes – or rather, 'the UK's leading innovator of residential later-life and care services'.

Carlauren had created a 'new private exchange token', and was going to use this 'breakthrough blockchain technology' to give residents of its care homes a 'safe and secure currency' to pay for their rooms and other services. My first reaction was: 'You can*not* be *serious!*' The idea that vulnerable elderly people – even the wealthy ones being targeted by this scheme – would be well served by having to acquire a cryptocurrency to pay for their care home rooms seemed ludicrous.

But when I got hold of Carlauren's founder and chief executive, Sean Murray, he assured me that he was completely serious. His plan was to create what he called the C-Coin, priced at £70: the cost of one night's accommodation – though not care – in one of his luxury care homes, or 'resorts', as he styled them. He was launching this currency with, you've guessed it, an Initial Coin Offering. There was a bonus safety mechanism: at any stage you could sell the £70 coins back to the company for £63, thereby limiting the risk of investing in cryptocurrency. He painted this as an innovative way of allowing well-off elderly people and their children to invest in their room for the long term – a kind of timeshare scheme which would then be tradeable, because the coins could be sold on an exchange. 'I wanted to crystallize the payment of the room for the foreseeable future,' he explained. He outlined a membership scheme whereby residents who were currently paying between £1,250 and £1,500 a week would buy their room with the tokens, and it would be an asset for their children after they died. 'We see an opportunity with family members that are obviously wisely aware of what's happening in the crypto market – that has an intrinsic value.'

When I expressed a few doubts, Mr Murray seemed surprised. He kept stressing that he was a visionary who was coming into the fusty old care industry and shaking things up. 'No one likes change, but we have to move with the times. Our younger generation will become older, and it takes visionaries such as myself to make these changes.'

To see how this story would play out I decided I needed to buy one of these C-Coins on the Carlauren exchange. I signed up for membership, and could immediately see that nearly all of the 500,000 coins were still available at a price of £70. Bizarrely, the exchange also listed a market price of £189 for the coins. Here's an opportunity, I thought, to make a speedy profit.

So I bought for £70, and immediately sold my coin for £189. Or so it seemed. The next day the £70 had gone from my bank account, but my sale was still marked on the exchange as pending. But strangely, moments after my purchase, a marketing email had popped into my inbox with an excited message:

We want to let you know that someone has just bought 1 C-Coins at £70 / 1 C-Coin.

The current market price of one C-Coin is **£189.0017** / 1 C-Coin.

The email, obviously triggered by my purchase, ended by asking, 'Is it time to buy or sell?' It looked to me like a deeply dishonest piece of marketing designed to make people think they could make a fast buck.

So I got back in touch with Sean Murray. He explained that this £189.0017 market price would only be available once all 500,000 coins had been sold. That price had been calculated using a formula so complex that I was unable to follow it, but he agreed that the wording on the exchange website needed to be clearer.

Further digging revealed that the Carlauren empire, far from being the leading player in the care industry painted by that original press release, was actually a newcomer, with at most a couple of homes actually caring for residents. The rest were a scattering of properties across the country which had been bought up for renovation, with the rooms sold off to investors on the promise of long-term returns. What's more, the very basic accounts published at Companies House suggested that this was a company with big liabilities, and might be in a parlous financial position.

Sensing that there was a lot more to come out about Carlauren and its plans to put elderly people on the blockchain, I wrote a long blogpost – after conversations with the BBC lawyer – headlined 'Crypto for care homes – really?' Then I sat back and waited to see what happened.

It didn't take long. By July one of Carlauren's care homes in Somerset had closed after staff complained they had not been paid for a month. Further investigation revealed that the company's one other care home was also closed.

Meanwhile, unhappy investors got in touch to tell me they had received a newsletter telling them that Carlauren was now getting out of the care business and would focus on hotel development. Further delving into the complex web of companies revealed that it included Carlauren Travel, which owned several luxury cars, and Carlauren Aviation, which had purchased a corporate jet.

After I had made several fruitless attempts to contact the visionary Sean Murray he eventually came back with a few answers to my many questions. Yes, he had told me that the business was well funded back in the spring but, 'due to market changes with third parties, our income changed.' As for the revolutionary cryptocurrency plan, that was 'on hold' but, rest assured, the buyback guarantee that would at least give me and other investors £63 for each and every £70 coin still stood. I wrote another long blogpost, this time with the headline 'Crypto for care homes – one bad idea'. After that I left the story alone – after all, it had been a fascinating excursion into the murky world of cryptocurrency schemes, but the troubles of a failing property business were not really the province of a technology correspondent.

You will not be surprised to hear what happened next. By the end of the year the Carlauren empire had collapsed into administration, with investors who had put £75 million behind Sean Murray's vision looking unlikely to scc their money again. The administrators turned up a sadly familiar story of lavish spending on cars, the aforementioned corporate jet and a couple of luxury homes.

A few months on, a *BBC North East* investigation revealed that a decade earlier Murray had been involved in a property scam in the United States. UK investors had been invited to buy homes in the ailing city of Detroit, with the promise of a decent return from tenants. But many of the properties, it turned out, were essentially derelict, and the investors, who had been shown misleading photos, were soon receiving no income. Confronted by the BBC at a second-hand car lot where he was working, Murray said he couldn't remember ten years ago.

As for my £70 C-Coin, it is stuck somewhere in cyberspace, and I think I am as likely to get it back as I am to get a refund of the BTC 0.017 I sent to Satoshi Nakamoto back in 2016. A pity, really, because at the time of writing the latter is worth about £127.

It might seem unfair to tarnish the whole cryptocurrency and blockchain scene with tales of dodgy characters and ridiculously unrealistic schemes. But in two decades of covering emerging technologies I have never come across any sector where the gap between what was promised and what was delivered has been so wide. Despite the continuing blizzard of marketing from PRs and consultants, I have yet to see anything to convince me that Bitcoin or similar currencies, distributed ledgers or smart contracts are going to create valuable new businesses or transform our lives for the better.

As 2020 dawned, it felt as though the public was tiring of the technology revolution.

New ideas, from cryptocurrencies to augmented reality, were failing to cut through, and, on the surface at least, it appeared that the pace of innovation was slowing. Smartphones and social media were still driving important changes in society, but people were becoming less clear that these changes were for the better. A series of scandals had weakened trust in the major technology companies, and there was growing appetite for regulation amongst politicians. When the UK internet and society think tank doteveryone published a survey early that year, it highlighted how hope in the positive power of technology had ebbed away. While 81 per cent of respondents felt the internet had improved their own lives, just 50 per cent felt optimistic about how technology would affect society in the future.

As for the tech companies, just 19 per cent of those surveyed believed the businesses designed their products and services with their best interests in mind, and 50 per cent felt that it was 'part and parcel' of being online that people would try to cheat or harm them in some way. Doteveryone's founder Martha Lane Fox, whom we met earlier, called on government, regulators and industry to 'listen to the concerns people voice and act urgently to create a digital future that's good for people and the planet.'

In the UK and in many other countries it had been a tempestuous few years, with divisions opening up on issues ranging from Brexit to the election of Donald Trump. Technology was increasingly seen as a malign force, driving people apart rather than bringing them together. But then a global crisis arrived like no other the world had seen for decades. It would shake politics and economics to their foundations, with no country untouched by the shockwaves. It would also provide an opportunity for us all to rethink our relationship with technology, which was to prove immensely valuable but equally dangerous in our time of need.

Part III

Tech in a Global Health Crisis

11

The Pandemic Arrives

At the beginning of January 2020 I made my way up into the loft of my West London home to begin work on this book, in what had been the teenage bedroom of my older child. I had the book fairly well mapped out in my head. I would start with the arrival of the social smartphone era and all the excitement and optimism that came with it, before charting how we all began to lose faith in this digital utopia, and then end with a personal and hopefully uplifting exploration of what technology could do to improve healthcare as I grappled with both Parkinson's and cancer of the eye. (In 2005 I had been given radiotherapy for a malignant melanoma behind my left eye, and from time to time needed more treatment when the tumour showed signs of growing again.)

But soon I had to rethink this final section, because of events that put both healthcare and the role of technology, for good and ill, front and centre for everyone, not just me. On 3 January, as I sat writing about the launch of the iPhone, a small story appeared on the BBC website. 'Chinese authorities,' it said, 'have launched an investigation into a mysterious viral pneumonia which has infected dozens of people in the central city of Wuhan. A total of 44 cases have been confirmed so far, 11 of which are considered "severe", officials said on Friday.'

I thought nothing of it. Well, in fact I didn't even read it, and I suspect neither did most people – even in the highest reaches of the

UK government, where all attention was focused on preparing for the end of the month and the country's departure from the EU.

Searching back through my email, the first mention of the virus comes on 21 January, in a daily list of business stories sent around my office. 'Shares in Chinese mask-makers and drug firms rise on Coronavirus outbreak,' read one story on the list. Again, I ignored it – what was a coronavirus, anyway?

But as January drew to a close the news from China did begin to seep through. On 27 January a BBC political correspondent sent round some copy on how the Prime Minister had responded when asked about evacuating British citizens from Wuhan. Mr Johnson, said the government, was 'doing everything we can to ensure that people who do come to this country are properly screened and checked if they've come from an area that is known to have the infection'. The emphasis was that this was a Chinese problem, and all we needed to do was make sure it stayed there. But that same day the medical director of Public Health England, Professor Yvonne Doyle, said she believed that coronavirus might already have arrived in the UK.

On 31 January came the first email to me with a virus-related tech story.

'Hi Rory', it read. 'My friend and I built a little app that enables to track [sic] the toll of the coronavirus in real-time.' I yawned. 'For the record,' it went on, 'we're both expats based in Taiwan, so we felt particularly concerned about the epidemic.'

Not a story, I thought. Anyway, it was my first day back in the office after four weeks off, and my attention was somewhere else. I was about to head off to California for ten days to make two editions of my radio programme *Tech Tent* and to attend a very high-powered conference. There were a few rumblings from the tech world about the impact of the virus – manufacturing in China was being disrupted, and there was even a faintly ridiculous rumour that Mobile World Congress, the huge industry shindig in Barcelona in late February, could be called off.

Yet I flew to California on 4 February with my mind focused on taking the temperature of Silicon Valley rather than a health crisis in China. While it was becoming clear that the coronavirus was becoming a major irritant to a technology industry hugely dependent on Chinese suppliers – and increasingly consumers   it was not going to have any greater impact in the West than the SARS epidemic had back in 2003. I had watched and enjoyed the dystopian thriller *Contagion*, about a global pandemic, but had viewed it as just another disaster movie with no relevance to my own life.

After landing in San Francisco we hurriedly interviewed a venture capitalist, the head of the Stanford University Medical School and a disgruntled Uber driver, as we put together an edition of *Tech Tent* headlined 'Has Silicon Valley Still Got It?' The extremely knowledgeable Uber driver gave us food for thought about the sustainability of a business model that saw companies making huge and growing losses but paying executives $43 million salaries while keeping the likes of him on minimum wage. But overall we still concluded that this was the place to be. The area, I wrote on my blog, still had a lot going for it: 'a huge pool of talent from around the world, vast amounts of venture capital, and a Californian confidence as sunny as the February weather has been for the last few days. Don't count Silicon Valley out just yet.' Then I headed off for the weekend to one of the dullest places on earth, Menlo Park, a sea of business parks that feels much like the M4 corridor to the west of London, except with palm trees and sunshine.

But I was bound for an exciting   nay, intimidating – event. something called a Social Sciences Foo Camp. This was a conference organized by the legendary Silicon Valley mover and shaker Tim O'Reilly, and it was hosted on the Facebook campus. I say conference – it was actually an 'unconference', with no fixed agenda, where people turn up and decide what they want to discuss. In this case those people were a collection of some of the finest minds in economics, psychology and political science, from the US and Europe, including two Nobel Prizewinners. There was the man who had invented the term 'filter bubble', a clutch of leading thinkers on AI, and a young quantum physicist who was now in 10 Downing Street advising Boris Johnson.

I found myself chatting to a pleasant American psychology professor called David Dunning, who revealed that he was an Arsenal fan, though, he confessed, no expert. I later realized that he was one of the duo that had formulated the Dunning–Kruger effect, an example of cognitive bias which says that the less you know, the more confident you are likely to be – whereas real experts know their limits.

Looking back at my notes on an incredibly stimulating weekend, where we discussed everything from the productivity paradox to the fake news phenomenon, one subject stands out by its absence. The coronavirus. While there was a session on health data and where the balance lay between privacy and public good – a topic suggested somewhat timidly by me – there was not a hint in this gathering of great minds that just six weeks later California, the UK and much of the rest of the world would be locked down as a global pandemic took hold.

But as I returned from Menlo Park to San Francisco to spend the last five days of the trip making another edition of *Tech Tent*, the virus was climbing up the agenda. More big tech companies had announced they were pulling out of Mobile World Congress and, having previously been convinced the event would still go ahead, I began to have my doubts. Reading the *San Francisco Chronicle* over breakfast, I came across an interview with a professor of infectious diseases at the University of California in Berkeley, who appeared to think that people were over-reacting to the threat from the coronavirus, with social media helping to spread panic. We caught the train over the Bay Bridge to interview Professor Lee Riley in his office on the Berkeley campus.

He seemed keen to downplay the seriousness of the epidemic. 'I think influenza is far more serious in terms of the number of cases that we've seen in the world and number of deaths caused by this infection.' He admitted that there was still a lot we did not know about the coronavirus, and said it was that uncertainty which drove the concerns and the fear. But should Mobile World Congress in

Barcelona be cancelled? No, that would be an over-reaction. Even if people were attending the show from China, he said, 'we have new ways to diagnose these types of infections very quickly and accurately, so that shouldn't be a concern.'

We did have to stop the interview at one point when the professor had a prolonged coughing fit. Seeing our concerned faces, the professor laughed – 'Don't worry,' he said. 'I haven't got the virus!' But a few days after our return from the United States, my producer Jat developed a hacking cough which took days to shake off. He never got a test, but we wondered afterwards whether the coronavirus had already been circulating in San Francisco.

We left Berkeley that afternoon somewhat reassured that our regular trip to Barcelona at the end of the month was still on, and that maybe the virus was not going to be such a big story after all. Over the next 48 hours all that changed.

The next day we went off to cover a major mobile phone launch. Samsung, the biggest player in the market, used to unveil its flagship phone at Mobile World Congress, but the previous year it had pre-empted the show with an event a week or so earlier. It was pulling the same trick this year with a launch at San Francisco's Palace of Fine Arts. In a typically glitzy presentation Samsung unveiled a series of 5G-capable smartphones and an eye-catching folding phone, the Z-Flip. But that was not the main thrust of the story we filed for TV and radio.

We had walked into the event past a thermal camera screening for anyone with a high temperature – a symptom of the coronavirus – and inside the hall masks and hand-cleansing gel were available. I directed our camera operator to get shots of people in the audience wearing masks – still an unusual sight in early February 2020 – and that was how our piece opened.

Millions of people around the world engage with stories about phone launches, and the Samsung event was a big deal, setting the scene for a year in which 5G was expected to become standard on phones and a hot topic in politics. We did shoot a separate show-and-tell video for the BBC website about the folding Z-Flip which got plenty of hits, but the fact that we led on the potential impact of the coronavirus on the industry showed which way the wind was blowing.

The following day news came through that the organizers of Mobile World Congress had bowed to the inevitable and cancelled it, after the withdrawal of so many of the leading tech firms. There was much talk of the huge damage to the economy of Barcelona caused by the loss of an event that draws over 100,000 people to the city. Had everyone panicked unnecessarily when there had been only a couple of cases of the virus recorded in Spain?

That same day an epidemiologist quoted in the *Guardian* said that the first case in London, involving someone who had travelled from China, was not something to get too worried about. 'We don't have enough evidence at this stage to say that it is spreading in London,' said Dr Michael Tildesley. 'We have had an introduction of the virus to London from an individual that has travelled from China but as yet, no reported human-to-human transmission as a result of this new case.' A global health expert, Dr Michael Head, was similarly reassuring: 'Risks to Londoners and UK residents remain low, though people should continue to keep an eye on guidance for the general public.' We returned to London from California aware that this was now going to be a big story for the technology industry, but still seeing it as something happening elsewhere, of little relevance to our own lives. Looking back, it is sobering to reflect how quickly that was to change.

On 3 March, just 51 cases of the virus had been confirmed in the UK, although there was worrying news from Italy, where there had been more than 2,500 cases and 80 deaths. I was selfishly focused on the situation in Italy, because I had a skiing holiday in the Dolomites planned for mid-March, and then a thirtieth wedding anniversary weekend in Venice in early April. For now, there appeared to be no reason why both trips should not go ahead. That day Boris Johnson spoke at a press conference about the precautions he was – or rather was not – taking: 'I was at a hospital the other night where I think there were . . . actually a few coronavirus patients, and I shook hands with everybody. You'll be pleased to know that I continue to shake hands.' Five weeks later, the Prime Minister was in the intensive care unit of St Thomas's Hospital, suffering the effects of what by then we knew as COVID-19.

But I cannot claim to have been any more careful about my own health. On 7 March I stood on a packed terrace at Griffin Park, home of my local football club, Brentford. As we beat Sheffield Wednesday 5–0 there were plenty of occasions where I ended up almost submerged in my fellow fans during enthusiastic goal celebrations.

That evening, the news came through that the Foreign Office was advising against travel to most of Northern Italy, as the death toll from the virus soared. That meant the trip to Venice was off, although curiously the Dolomites region was not included in the travel advisory, so my skiing holiday – just a week away – appeared to be unaffected. Suddenly, though, that was looking rather unappealing, so the closure of the ski lifts and the abrupt termination of the season two days later came as something of a relief.

The following week I commuted daily on packed Tube trains to my office in New Broadcasting House. It turned out to be the last few days I was to spend there for many months. Much of my work that week was occupied with a story about health – not what was rapidly turning into a global pandemic, but a very personal matter.

It was eighteen months since I had first started noticing during a holiday in Italy that I was dragging my right foot while walking, and just over a year since I had been diagnosed with Parkinson's disease. After the initial shock, I had grown determined to get something positive out of my situation by exploring the condition, and the part technology could play in searching for a cure and treating the symptoms.

I had got in touch with a company called Medopad, which I had first visited in October 2018, just a few months before my diagnosis. This fast-growing medical technology business was doing interesting work collecting information from smartphones and wearable devices and then getting machine learning algorithms to spot patterns in the data. It was working with the giant Chinese technology company Tencent on a project to try to use artificial intelligence to diagnose Parkinson's disease and monitor the progress of the condition. On that first visit to Medopad's offices high in London's Millbank Tower, we found the research team filming one of their Chinese collaborators opening and closing the fingers of one hand, stiffness in these kinds of movements being one of the symptoms of Parkinson's.

As we filmed him being filmed, I looked on, absent-mindedly opening and closing my fingers. I was beginning to suspect that I might have the condition, and wondered about asking them to film me, then thought better of the idea.

When I returned to Medopad in December 2019 I asked the founder, Dan Vahdat, whom I had interviewed the year before, whether he had noticed anything that suggested I might have a special interest in Parkinson's. 'I don't think we noticed anything specifically,' he said. 'But – and it's weird for me to tell you this – I had this intuition that I wanted to get you to do the test.'

The project had moved on, and there was now a clinical trial under way. Some people with Parkinson's had been given a smartphone app, which their relatives or carers had to use to film them doing not just the hand-clenching but a dozen or so other exercises. It was all about trying to give doctors a more fine-grained view of how Parkinson's disease was progressing in patients, Dan Vahdat explained.

> We think this technology can help to quantify the disease. And if you can . . . it means you can see how the disease progresses. It gives you lots of opportunities in terms of treatment adjustments, interventions at the right time, potentially screening a larger cohort of patients with the technology in ways that were not possible before.

That made me think about how my own treatment was progressing. Shortly after my diagnosis, the consultant treating me had gone through the pros and cons of medication. The benefits were that drugs could provide relief from the symptoms, though they would not stop the disease in its tracks. The downside was that there could be side-effects, and starting too early on a drug might mean that its impact lessened over the years.

We had decided to go ahead, and I'd been prescribed Sinemet, one of the most common Parkinson's drugs, in the form of two tablets taken three times a day. While some patients report instant effects shortly after taking the drug, which then wear off, leaving them urgently needing their next dose, that was not my experience. In fact, I struggled to notice any difference in my quite mild symptoms, although the foot-dragging did appear to have got marginally worse over time. I was only seeing my consultant once every four months, and each time we discussed altering my prescription, but it was hard for me to quantify my symptoms.

Dan Vahdat said this was a great example of the kind of issue the prototype app was trying to address. 'We think you will end up having a more continuous observation via machine, and the doctors can look at it remotely. And with that they will be able to adjust your treatment if needed, because potentially right now you're either overdosing or underdosing by default.'

While the trial was nearing its end, Medopad agreed that I could get hold of the app and try it out. So for the next couple of months one member of my family would film me going through the exercises – clenching my fist, walking back and forth across a room, getting up from a chair, writing my name down three times, drawing a spiral, and so on. The idea was that these little videos would all be uploaded to Medopad's cloud, and then the AI researchers and the doctors at King's College Hospital who were the other collaborators in the project would crunch all the data and come up with something clever.

The trouble was that, as the weeks went past, and we kept uploading the videos, there was no feedback, no visible output for the input of anyone on the trial. Was it generating useful results that would improve treatment? Maybe, but we simply did not know. In any case, calibrating the way existing drugs might be administered was all very well, but I was more interested in finding out about research that could lead to new drugs, and even a possible cure for this condition that afflicts so many people and curtails so many lives.

I had become involved in fundraising for Parkinson's UK, a relatively small but really effective charity with a big interest in research, and I had learned of a number of projects on which it and other charities were collaborating with artificial intelligence researchers. One involved a company I had already encountered, Benevolent AI, one of many hoping that healthcare could benefit from recent advances in machine learning techniques. The aim, the two organizations said in a statement unveiling their partnership, was 'to identify at least three currently available medicines that can be repurposed to address Parkinson's, and two brand-new ways to treat the condition with new drugs.' Rather depressingly, the statement also pointed out that there had been no major breakthroughs in the treatment of Parkinson's for over 50 years. That made me all the more determined to get involved with research that could help both me and others.

And in that week in the middle of March, just before everything stopped, there came an opportunity. A few weeks earlier, Parkinson's UK had invited me, along with several other people with the condition, to visit a laboratory at West London's Hammersmith Hospital. This was the home of the Parkinson's UK Brain Bank, the only one of its kind in the world and a vital resource in research.

We put on white coats and proceeded into the dissection room for one of the most electrifying demonstrations I have ever witnessed – outshining perhaps even Steve Jobs' unveiling of the iPhone. Another Steve, the head of the lab, Professor Steve Gentleman, took a brain out of a white plastic tub and began to dissect it.

As he did so, he explained the evidence of Parkinson's disease and other conditions he was coming across, and why it was so important that people like the 89-year-old woman whose medical story he was telling continued to leave their brains for research. Later, one of Professor Gentleman's colleagues described how, during his research for his doctorate at the Brain Bank, he had spotted the build-up of toxic iron in the brains of people with Parkinson's. This had fed into the development of a drug designed to remove the iron, which was currently going through clinical trials in the UK and France, with initial results suggesting it might slow the progress of the disease.

The charity had not brought us here just for a day out. It was soon to launch its first appeal in ten years for donors to the Brain Bank charity, seeking both people who had the condition and those who did not. A decade ago the broadcaster Jeremy Paxman had been among those to sign up. Now the charity wanted us to spread the word, and to think about becoming donors ourselves. The appeal was going to be launched on 16 March, and I decided that I could have a go at selling this as a story for television.

By then, the news agenda was concentrated ever more closely on the coronavirus, but I managed to convince *BBC Breakfast* that this would make an interesting film for them. There was one condition: they wanted it to be a very personal story, centred on my decision about whether I wanted to leave my own brain for this vital research.

So I found myself back at the Hammersmith Hospital in the dissection room with Steve Gentleman, plus a cameraman and a producer. Before he started cutting into the brain he was going to examine on camera, the professor handed it to me. I stood there marvelling at its weight, and at how strange it was that I did not feel squeamish – but also wondering whether a breakfast television audience would feel the same.

Steve Gentleman is one of those rare scientists who knows how to communicate a story in simple but precise language. As he began his dissection of the brain of an 84-year-old woman who had signed a consent form, he quickly found what he had been looking for. 'Lo and behold, this is entirely consistent with quite a long course of Parkinson's,' he said.

What had he spotted?

He explained that it was more a case of what he had not seen: a black line in a part of the brainstem called the *substantia nigra*, which represented dopamine cells. 'This lady has lost nearly all of those cells.'

The key thing we do know about Parkinson's is that it is caused by a deficiency of dopamine, the substance that sends messages from the brain to the rest of the body to control movement. I stretched out my right hand with its slight tremor, and put it to the professor that those cells might be disappearing from my brain too. He nodded.

As the dissection continued, I asked a few questions about the brain donor scheme, and why I should consider being part of it. I had my professional hat on, listening out for a 15-second soundbite that I could use in my TV report. Then he said this. 'These are invaluable, these brains. I have huge respect for people who make this commitment. It's a personal choice, but this is what makes us human. We are altruistic: we want to help other people.'

It was perfect – but his words packed such an emotional punch that I suddenly found myself close to tears.

After a short break, we decided we had enough shots of the dissection room, and went outside to get a final sequence: an interview with Parkinson's UK about the donor scheme, and a shot of me signing the form to become a brain donor.

Over the years, my TV reports for news programmes have rarely been longer than two and a half minutes – in exceptional circumstances an editor might allow you to go to three, though only after a tough negotiation. But the output editor of *Breakfast* on 16 March was in an exceptionally generous mood. My report, featuring Steve Gentleman's line about altruism and me getting choked up in response, ran for more than four and a half minutes, and was the most personal piece of journalism I had ever done.

What was really extraordinary in retrospect was that it got on air at all that day, on a programme otherwise almost exclusively devoted to the coronavirus crisis. By now football and many other spectator sports had been cancelled, the May local elections had been postponed for a year, and panic buying had stripped supermarkets of toilet rolls, pasta and other commodities suddenly deemed to be essentials. That evening, the Prime Minister told the nation that we had to take drastic new measures to combat the virus. We needed to start working from home wherever possible, and to avoid pubs, clubs and theatres, although they were not actually ordered to close. A couple of days later Boris Johnson's father Stanley was quoted as saying, 'I'll go to a pub if I need to go to a pub.'

But that evening's announcement did include something that would certainly prevent me from going in search of alcoholic refreshment. Certain people at increased risk of severe illness from coronavirus needed to be 'particularly stringent in following social-distancing measures'. That included people with chronic neurological conditions such as Parkinson's. I would definitely be working from home, with no clue as to when I would be allowed to head into my office at New Broadcasting House again. But I was only a week ahead of everyone else. On 23 March, in another prime ministerial broadcast, Boris Johnson told us all to Stay at Home, Protect the NHS and Save Lives. A country in lockdown was about to find out just how vital technology that we had begun to take for granted could be.

One morning at the end of March, a week into the full lockdown, I sat in my new base in the loft contemplating how quickly we had all adapted to these extraordinary circumstances. During that week, I had soon developed a fixed routine. Before 7 each morning I set out for my walk with the dog, my one permitted daily outing for exercise. I got into the habit of taking a picture each time and posting it on Instagram just to mark that another day had passed in lockdown. A British journalist based in Hong Kong sent me a message saying he now looked out for it each day as a reminder of home.

At 0820 I had my first video conference call of the day with BBC colleagues, followed by another at 0920 and a third at 10. Downstairs my wife, an economics professor, was also on endless video calls, both organizing the public policy institute she ran and getting involved in various projects to chart the economic effects of the pandemic. Every now and then she would call upstairs to ask me to shut my door, because my noisy and sometimes profane conversations with my fellow journalists were disturbing her more sedate and highbrow interactions with academics and civil servants. One afternoon she complained that, while she was chairing a UN panel, I could be heard shouting 'You fucking idiots!' In my defence, I was watching a House of Commons Select Committee and, over the course of an hour, the MPs had failed to ask the witness the key question I needed answered to move a story on.

Like just about everyone else I knew, my video-conferencing platform of choice was Zoom, a service that before the lockdown had been familiar only to those in the business world. In December 2019 10 million people a day took part in Zoom meetings. By April 2020 that had leaped to 300 million, with most apparently unconcerned by warnings that it was insecure. There were numerous accounts of 'Zoom bombing', where outsiders crashed meetings or even interrupted them by screening pornography, until the company made it easier to lock them down. Soon, even Boris Johnson's Cabinet meetings were being held on Zoom.

For me it became the vital infrastructure needed to organize my weekly radio programme *Tech Tent*. We conducted interviews with people in the United States, India and all sorts of other places via the service. The sound quality was often not great, but we asked guests to record their end of the conversation on a smartphone and then email it to us. Then on a Friday morning we would record the whole programme on a Zoom call, with me and a BBC tech desk colleague debating the big stories of the week while producer Jat Gill listened in. Again, we would each record separately into a smartphone or digital recorder, and then send it all to Jat at his home just outside London. He would then edit and assemble the whole programme on an iPad before uploading it onto the BBC's servers.

But Zoom soon became vital to leisure as well as business. My Saturday morning Pilates class, an essential part of my fitness regime, was now conducted over the video-conferencing platform, with the teacher probably able to monitor how well her eight or ten customers were doing more easily via her laptop than when we had been in her studio.

My wife and I realized that our Sunday evening ritual of walking to the houses of nearby friends for a drink and a chat about the week was no longer allowed – a big hole in our social life. But it quickly became a Zoom event too, and almost as good, although lacking the easy to-and-fro of real-world conversation – and we had to provide our own wine and cake.

Of course, life in lockdown was not all about Zoom. While I was not allowed to go filming or, like a few colleagues, to head into New Broadcasting House and appear in the studio, I was still managing to appear live on BBC news programmes. My camera in my loft office was an iPhone on a mini tripod, with cables plugged in for an external mic and some earphones. The engineers back at base would call me up via Skype and put me through to the studio. I did have to remember to slip on a formal shirt, but I could still broadcast in shorts – after all, the shot was carefully framed to feature only my top half.

Our day started and finished with a FaceTime call with our son and his wife and our one-year-old granddaughter. My piano teacher preferred to conduct our weekly lesson via a WhatsApp video call, and communication with friends and family ranged across everything from Facebook to Instagram to direct messages on Twitter.

And we were not atypical. Every kind of activity, from pub quizzes to ballet classes to bridge clubs, moved to online platforms. New stars were born: the Joe Wicks daily exercise class on YouTube drew huge audiences, while TikTok became the platform of choice for breakthrough comedians like Sarah Cooper, an American who lip synced to the ramblings of Donald Trump, and the UK's Meggie Foster, who worked a similar trick with Boris Johnson.

With theatres and cinemas closed, use of streaming platforms like Netflix, Amazon Prime and Apple TV rocketed. The movie industry postponed some major releases, but opted to put others online to buy or rent straight away. For theatre, ballet and classical music life was much harder, though the National Theatre began to stream classic productions on YouTube, while for 52 consecutive evenings the pianist Igor Levit used Twitter and YouTube to perform works by Beethoven, Bach, Nina Simone and Billy Joel from his Berlin home. And if that was not to your liking, every Friday evening you could watch Sophie Ellis-Bextor's kitchen disco as she danced in a sparkly dress while her five children played around her feet.

Meanwhile, with schools also closed, parents found themselves in the unenviable role of supply teachers, trying to deliver education from the kitchen table. But again technology came to their aid, with many schools using platforms like Google Classroom or Microsoft Teams to put teachers in touch with millions of pupils. Lockdown did, however, highlight a big digital divide, both in terms of access to technology such as laptops, and in the provision of online learning. In May a report from the Institute of Education warned that overall the amount of schoolwork being done at home was low, and there were big variations both geographically and between social groups. Children in the north-east of England were being given about a third as much work to complete at home as those in the South-East. Thirty-one per cent of private schools provided four or more live online lessons daily, compared to just 6 per cent of state schools. And while just about every private school pupil had access to a computer at home, one in five children getting free school meals – a measure of a low-income household – were in homes without any computer. For school students at key stages there was particular anxiety, with exams on which their future depended being cancelled. Later, there were huge rows about A-Level and GCSE grades calculated by algorithms: probably the first time algorithmic bias entered the national conversation.

In summary, lockdown was hard, desperately hard for many people, whether families with parents still trying to work while looking after children or those marooned at home alone. But the technology of 2020 did make a big difference to how we got through those long weeks when everything we took for granted – work, school, our social lives – was put on hold.

As I sat thinking about this that late March morning, at a time when I was in the early stages of writing this book, I wondered how we might have coped with this pandemic if it had arrived before the smartphone era.

Imagine that COVID-19 had been COVID-05, sweeping around the world in 2005. Two years before the launch of the iPhone, most people in the UK and other Western countries had a mobile phone, but it was used almost exclusively for talking and texting. Those activities would have certainly boomed during a pandemic, but this was the era before apps. So much of what we use our phones for today would not have been possible.

Take social media, for instance. The very term would have been greeted with quizzical looks, even though many people were rediscovering old school friends via the British site Friends Reunited, which was bought by ITV in 2005. Facebook was a year old, but was still an American college phenomenon, only arriving in UK universities in the autumn of that year. Neither Instagram nor WhatsApp had been invented, let alone Snapchat and TikTok, although YouTube was born that summer, and Twitter would come along the following year.

Back then, for just about everyone who was not a Blackberry-toting executive, the internet and email were something to be experienced on an office or home computer rather than on the move. In the UK, about 8 million households had a broadband connection, allowing their computers to access the internet at speeds of up to 10 megabits per second, while 7 million homes were still crawling along at dial-up speeds. That meant that all sorts of services that would later prove vital during the lockdown were only just getting off the ground.

While Skype had been started by Swedish entrepreneurs in 2003, it was for cheap internet telephony, and video calls would not be added to the service until 2006. In fact, the whole idea of video telephones, first demonstrated at the 1964 World's Fair, had yet to become a reality – at least for anyone but a few people in businesses able to afford high-end video-conferencing services.

No Zooming back then, no communing with friends using apps such as House Party, no office gossip circulating via WhatsApp or Slack or Facebook Messenger or countless other services. As for entertainment, instead of a plethora of online services from Netflix to Spotify to the online gaming platform Twitch, we would have had to get by with good, old-fashioned broadcast TV and radio, while raiding our collections of CDs and videotapes.

Without well-developed online learning platforms, and with quite a high proportion of children having neither a computer nor a home broadband connection, delivering schooling would have been even tougher. Schools might have put a few worksheets in the post, but making sure homework was completed would have been down to parents.

While shutting down the airlines, most shops and much of the services sector did enormous damage to the economy in 2020, it would have been even worse 15 years earlier. During the coronavirus pandemic, many people whose work involved commuting to an office found that they could operate at least as effectively from home, a development that is likely to have lasting consequences for patterns of work and transport use. Maybe that would still have been the case in 2005, but without smartphones, video-conferencing and fast broadband connections it is difficult to see how that would have worked well for many people. It would certainly have been much harder for me to broadcast from my loft, or for us to put together an entire radio programme without going into the office.

As we've seen in earlier chapters, we had very quickly become accustomed to the tools of the social smartphone era, even blasé about them, and mistrustful of the technology giants that provided them. Now we embraced them as never before, and tried to make sure elderly relatives had access to them. The debate about the digital divide between young and old, town and country, acquired a new urgency as it became clear that fast broadband was now an essential service – and, according to some, a better destination for public funds than a high-speed rail route. The wave of enthusiasm for digital technology which in the UK had peaked around the time of the London Olympics in 2012 had faded as we'd grown more and more worried about what smartphones and social media were doing to society and to us as individuals. Now that switchback ride between hopes for the technology and fear of it seemed to have taken us on another upward path, as the virus made us fall back in love with it.

As for those big bad technology companies, the heat seemed to be off, for a while at least. Amazon might have seemed the enemy of the high street – and independent bookshops in particular – and its employment practices had attracted plenty of criticism, but its unrivalled expertise in logistics now made it vital in at least keeping economics ticking over. The UK government even had it delivering coronavirus home-testing kits, and the company's AWS cloud computing division allowed all sorts of services to cope with a surge in traffic.

Microsoft and Google also proved their worth in the cloud, with Microsoft's CEO Satya Nadella marvelling that his firm had seen two years' worth of digital transformation in just two months as customers adapted to life in a pandemic. As the world began to lock down in early March and more people started to work from home, both companies began offering for free some of the services which enterprises had been paying for – a savvy marketing move which also made them look generous.

Even Facebook, in the crosshairs of regulators and politicians from both left and right at the beginning of the year, seemed to feel the pressure ease as even bigger audiences flocked to use its services. Its chief executive Mark Zuckerberg made it clear from the beginning that he took the coronavirus seriously, sending staff home, backing state plans for tight restrictions on movement, even when some other tech leaders grumbled, and unveiling plans to combat misinformation about the virus. In March the *Washington Post* wrote that Zuckerberg and his senior colleagues 'see the pandemic as a chance to prove the service's value to a wary public after it has been clouded by past mistakes'.

As we will find out later, that did not quite work out as planned but, whatever the popular view of the tech companies, the stock market continued to love them. After a market meltdown in March as investors panicked about a virus-induced economic depression, it was the tech giants that led an almost insane recovery in the mood. By June, shares in Amazon, Apple and Facebook were hitting new all-time highs, while Google's owner Alphabet was up nearly 40 per cent from its March low point. Meanwhile Zoom, a company few had heard of at the beginning of the year, was for a while worth more than the seven biggest airlines combined. In the UK, the online retailer and robotics specialist Ocado was suddenly worth twice as much as the aero engine maker Rolls-Royce, for decades Britain's most successful engineering business.

Amidst the huge disruption caused by a global health crisis the technology of the smartphone era was galloping forward once again, leaving the twentieth century's pioneers gasping by the roadside. But pleasing volatile investors was one thing. Proving that you could make a serious contribution to the battle against the biggest threat faced by most countries for decades was quite another.

12

The App That Could Tame COVID

We heard earlier about that growing sense of disappointment in the achievements of the technology industry in the smartphone era, summed up by Peter Thiel's line about being promised flying cars and getting 140 characters. While the way we lived in 2020 looked on the surface to have been transformed by the revolution in connectivity the smartphone had brought with it, that was not reflected in economic growth, and in one key statistic in particular.

Increasing productivity, or what we get out for what we put in – the number of cars produced per worker hour, for example – is the key to improving our standard of living. It is advances in technology which boost productivity and so make us all better off, as we saw in the second half of the twentieth century. So if the smartphone and the internet really were the big advances in technology we thought them to be, then that story should have been reflected in the productivity numbers.

As 2019 drew to a close, however, the Royal Statistical Society chose as its statistic of the decade UK productivity growth of 0.3 per cent per annum. This very poor number, it had decided, said a lot about the state we were in. The judging panel emphasized that this was the worst period for productivity growth since the early nineteenth century, comparing it to the 2 per cent annual growth which had been the long-term average.

In mitigation, economic historians noted that technology revolutions often take time to feed through into productivity statistics, for two reasons. First, because we find it difficult to measure the output of new gadgets – a 2020 iPhone is a much more powerful computer than the original 2007 version, but the statisticians who measure its contribution to GDP will treat it much the same – and secondly because it takes time for us to reorganize the way we work around the new technology.

Now, for the tech utopians, the pandemic that arrived in 2020 provided an opportunity to show that the new tools really could make a difference in the most fundamental way. The discovery that millions could work from home effectively, and that much business travel was unnecessary, for example, would at last bring a productivity revolution to many service industries. But far more exciting was the idea that technology could play a part in both controlling and beating the coronavirus. Tech leaders from Bill Gates to Google's Sundar Pichai and Apple's Tim Cook were eager to enlist the industry's data-mining skills and vast brainpower in helping policymakers to tackle this huge challenge.

The priority, of course, was to find a vaccine, and this was the job of the established pharmaceutical companies, not the tech giants.

Or was it?

The virus had come along just as the boom in artificial intelligence was at its peak, with many of the leading lights focusing on healthcare as the area where their research could make big breakthroughs. At a clutch of AI conferences the previous year I'd heard many a speaker talk of accelerating the process of drug discovery as the holy grail.

Developing, testing and bringing to market a new drug is a hugely costly business that can take well over a decade. If machine learning techniques could help identify new compounds much more quickly and then accelerate the testing process, that could save both money and lives. Now the apostles of AI had the most urgent challenge imaginable: help find a vaccine for COVID-19 before it killed even more people and wrought untold damage on the world economy.

There was an extraordinary advance in 2020, and once again it came from Google's DeepMind. Demis Hassabis and his team solved one of biology's greatest mysteries, predicting how a protein folds, in order to understand its three-dimensional shape. For decades scientists had been puzzling over ways of accelerating a process which could take many months of work in a lab. Now DeepMind showed that its deep learning program AlphaFold could complete the same task in hours, an achievement described as truly remarkable by independent scientists. It promised to advance understanding of diseases such as Parkinson's, thought to be linked to proteins being distorted into the wrong shapes, and so make treatments for them a lot easier to discover. But it was December by the time this achievement was unveiled, too late to help in the battle against COVID-19. Older techniques had been used to create three effective vaccines at a remarkable speed.

Back at the beginning of the year, there was a more immediate way in which the technology industry thought its skills were relevant: one in which governments around the world were eager to seek help. As every country strove to track the virus and limit its spread, the realization dawned that most of their citizens were carrying with them a communications device which could play a vital role.

The smartphone had already shown that it could change just about everything: the way we communicated and shopped, travelled and managed our finances, organized our romantic lives and got our news. Whatever you wanted to do, there was an app for that. So why not an app to stop the coronavirus from spreading?

From early on, China and other Asian countries had used smartphones to track their citizens and make sure they were not breaking quarantine. On *Tech Tent* we interviewed a young Taiwanese man who, on returning home from a stay in Europe, had been told that he needed to be quarantined for 14 days and warned that his phone would be satellite-tracked. Then one morning his phone ran out of battery, and 45 minutes later the police came knocking at his door. They wanted to check that he was still at home, not evading quarantine.

But it was Singapore which had the most ambitious plan, launching an app which used a smartphone's Bluetooth connection to monitor how people infected with the virus came into contact with others. This was a brand-new idea, featuring untested technology, but promised to provide a fast and comprehensive way to trace the contacts of anyone who fell sick. Countries around the world decided they needed to follow the same route. That included the UK, where a team had been assembled to build an app shortly before the country went into lockdown. I found out about this in late March not long after I had retreated to my loft, and from then on spent months immersed in the tale of a project which seemed to encapsulate the troubled relationship between the 'move fast and break things' technology industry, the more cautious public health officials, and a government desperate to find a way out of a crisis which it knew was not going well.

A few days after we had gone into lockdown my phone pinged, and I found a text message from a senior figure in the UK tech industry. This person, who had run successful tech businesses for more than 20 years and also acted as a government adviser, told me they were 'helping the NHS on a very substantial project that will launch in days and potentially save hundreds of thousands of British lives'. Very intriguing, I thought.

When I called to find out more, I learned that the project was a mobile phone app that would help trace the contacts of anyone who had been infected with the virus. But the tech luminary obviously had a somewhat misguided view, both of my expertise in app development and of my role at the BBC, suggesting that I might act as a consultant to the project. I gently explained that as a reporter I could not have such a role even in what felt at that stage like wartime circumstances, but I was very interested in knowing as much as possible about this important story.

My contact saw the sense in this. From then on I got great access to the gripping tale of what at first seemed to be a heroic attempt by technologists to lead the fight against the virus using the device that had already changed the way we communicated. Finally, the smartphone was going to prove that it really did rank with penicillin and electric power as an innovation that could actually change our lives for the better!

It had been at a meeting on Saturday, 7 March, at the Department of Health, that the project was born. As well as civil servants and public health experts, scientists from Oxford's Big Data Institute and, intriguingly, representatives of a division of GCHQ gathered in the office of the Permanent Secretary. 'The spooks and Oxford had independently come to the same conclusion: that an app-based system could actually snuff out the virus,' one of those present remembers. The wheels were then set in motion, a team was assembled, and a software developer, VMware Pivotal, was hired to work on the app.

As I set to work to understand the story, I got hold of a PowerPoint presentation which started with a slide illustrating the four aims of the project:

- Stop or flatten the epidemic
- Control the flow of patients into hospitals
- Help people return to normal life
- Gather secondary data for use by the NHS and strategic leaders

Now, I was already aware that many governments around the world were using mobile phones in the battle to contain the virus, some of them in very intrusive ways. That story of the Taiwanese man in quarantine was just one example. Taiwan was one of a number of Asian countries that had been successful in controlling the virus, with few complaints from citizens about the methods employed. In South Korea too there had been little opposition to what was effectively a programme of mass surveillance. The government collected data from mobile phone masts, from credit card transactions and from CCTV to map with precision the movements of people who were infected with the virus. 'They have taken information methods that are normally used by law enforcement to catch tax evaders or to track criminals, and they've repurposed those for public health use,' Justin Fendos, a professor of cell biology at Dongseo University in the South Korean city of Busan, explained to me.

A lot of this information was made available via text alerts to people's phones and on public websites. You could go online and see that case 10932 had visited various cafés, restaurants and offices over a couple of days before receiving a positive test result and being transferred to a hospital. Presumably, it would not be too difficult for colleagues and relatives of patient 10932 to work out the person behind the number. The populations of both Taiwan and South Korea had experience of the SARS epidemic, and their countries had been run by authoritarian governments until relatively recently, so perhaps it is not surprising that they did not resist such an intrusive approach to fighting the virus.

Those kinds of methods were never going to be acceptable in the UK or many other Western countries. But Singapore, often seen as a place whose government was a little too keen on exerting control over its citizens, was winning praise for its TraceTogether app, which looked less intrusive than many.

It took advantage of a phone's Bluetooth connection to record contacts between app users. Then, when someone tested positive for the virus, anyone who had been in close enough contact with them over the previous few days would get a notification from the app telling them to go into quarantine. It was this Bluetooth method that was adopted in the UK and in many other countries around the world as a potential magic bullet that might identify COVID-19 carriers before they infected anyone else.

In my early conversations with the team at NHSX (the department of the NHS in charge of new technology) they were keen to stress the academic underpinning of their approach, pointing me to an interview two Oxford academics had given to *Channel 4 News* just before the lockdown. Professor Christophe Fraser of the Oxford Big Data Institute and Dr David Bonsall from the John Radcliffe Hospital were interviewed after a package which suggested they were advocating an approach similar to the very intrusive one used in China, something they did not deny. Perhaps that was because their expertise was not in smartphone technology but in epidemiology. They went on to stress that an app could reduce the frequency with which the virus was transmitted, and even reverse the epidemic. Months later, Dr David Bonsall told me what their thinking had been back then. 'Very fast contact tracing was likely to be essential. And smartphones have the technological capability to speed up that process.'

It soon became clear that Christophe Fraser, who had been at that first meeting at the Department of Health, was going to be hugely influential in the direction the NHS project would take, especially as he was available to talk about it on radio and TV, when the developers and managers taking decisions about it were not. He appeared keen for the app to go beyond mere contact tracing, and provide data that would be of use in understanding the nature of the pandemic both now and after it was over, the fourth point on that PowerPoint I'd seen. This was later to prove controversial.

It is worth pausing here to look at how contact tracing works. I learned something about this practice, which goes back centuries, when I was trying to find out how the people being recruited in May to be part of a large-scale manual contact tracing programme were being trained. Meeting resistance from the Department of Health, which did not want to show me what were apparently pretty sparse teaching materials, I enrolled on an online course run by Johns Hopkins University in the United States.

This proved to be an exhausting but enlightening experience: eight hours of absorbing, really well-produced videos featuring actors playing the parts of contact tracers and the people they had to call, followed by a whole series of very tricky multiple-choice questions. I emerged gratified with my 95 per cent pass rate in the final exam and a certificate confirming that I was now a qualified contact tracer.

But more significantly I learned some key lessons about COVID-19, and how short a window there was to track down people who might have come into contact with the virus. One slide told the story. It depicted an encounter between two people, one of whom was already infected but was not yet showing symptoms. It then showed what was called a 'five-day window of opportunity' before that second person themselves became infectious. The implication was that you needed the first person to get tested the moment they got symptoms, and the second person – their contact – to be reached as soon as possible after that and told to go into quarantine so the chain of infection could be broken. The other lesson was that telling someone they had to do that was a very sensitive task, involving great communication skills and an understanding of privacy and data protection issues. It did not sound like a job that could be done by an app notification.

But here was the problem for the UK back in March 2020. We had neither widely available rapid testing, nor a functioning manual contact tracing programme. That, apparently, was why the government got so excited about the idea that an app could do the whole job. Not only might it offer a way to identify people who would be missed by a manual contact tracing programme – the person standing next to you on a crowded bus – but, a couple of months before the decision was made to recruit thousands of human beings to do the job, it was also the only game in town.

Even back then, as ministers urged the NHSX team to pursue this project with maximum speed and never mind the cost, technology experts were urging caution. That was because the whole idea of Bluetooth contact tracing apps was brilliant in theory, but had yet to be shown to work in practice.

Another slide in the PowerPoint presentation about the NHSX app showed what was called a 'controlled database of proximity events': a record of times when two devices had been recorded as being within 2 metres of each other for a certain time, as measured by the Bluetooth Low Energy protocol. Then, when one of the devices was recorded as belonging to someone who had a positive test, that central database would send an alert to the other phone to warn its owner to go into quarantine. But this slide highlighted two fundamental issues that were to dog the project. A centralized NHS database holding large amounts of sensitive information about citizens' contacts with one another was going to set alarm bells ringing among privacy campaigners and data protection specialists. And using Bluetooth was going to be tricky for all sorts of reasons.

At first sight, it appeared more attractive than using the GPS sensor on a phone, which would not work deep within buildings or if you were on an underground train. What is more, it was felt that Bluetooth would seem less privacy-invasive than GPS, which most people would understand as a location-tracking system. The idea here was to track proximity to other phones, not geographical location. Bluetooth, familiar to people as a way of linking a smartphone to headphones or swapping photos between devices, could drain a phone's battery quite quickly, but Bluetooth Low Energy was a variant which seemed to mitigate that issue. There was, however, a lot of doubt about just how accurately it could measure distance. Professor Alan Woodward, a cybersecurity specialist from the University of Surrey who provided advice to the app team at various points, says he made one thing clear from the start: 'It's never going to be perfect, because it's Bluetooth.' Expecting it to tell you with some reliability whether two phones were within 2 metres of one another was going to be quite a stretch.

Jon Crowcroft, a Cambridge University computing professor who had actually made a Bluetooth contact tracing app 12 years before during the H1N1 virus outbreak, was also realistic about what the project might achieve. But he had assumed it would just be a supplement to a full manual programme. 'I didn't realize how much the government was adrift on the manual contact tracing. Having worked with epidemiologists and public health people twelve years ago, I assumed we still had in place the local contact tracing that's used when there are things like university or school outbreaks of meningitis.'

Moreover, if the app was going to be the key method of contact tracing, then it would have to be downloaded by a lot of people. Early on, Christophe Fraser talked about the need for 60 per cent of the UK population to install the app if it was to stop COVID-19 in its tracks – and later on he made it clear that amounted to something like 80 per cent of all smartphone users. A very tall order, especially when it emerged that, once downloaded, the app might affect a phone's performance.

This was due to another issue with Bluetooth. Apple and Google, makers of the two dominant mobile operating systems, iOS and Android, were very cautious about allowing apps to keep using Bluetooth when they were running in the background. And soon there was worrying news from Singapore, where users seemed reluctant to install TraceTogether because it needed to be kept open on the phone all the time, draining the battery.

That, however, did not seem to worry the man who had overall charge of the UK's app, Secretary of State for Health Matt Hancock. On 12 April, at the regular Downing Street press conference, on a day when he also had to announce more than 650 deaths from the virus, he unveiled what he described as the next step in the battle against COVID-19. 'If you become unwell with the symptoms of coronavirus,' he explained, 'you can securely tell this new NHS app, and the app will then send an alert anonymously to other app users that you've been in significant contact with over the past few days, even before you had symptoms, so that they know and can act accordingly.' He also promised that all data would be handled securely and ethically, and went on, 'We're already testing this app and, as we do this, we're working closely with the world's leading tech companies and renowned experts in clinical safety and digital ethics so that we can get this right.'

So if it was already being tested, it seemed the project was quite advanced – though one of the advisers to the app team thought that perhaps the Health Secretary, who had launched his own app to publicize his work as an MP a couple of years earlier, was letting his natural enthusiasm get the better of him. 'Matt Hancock is a great technophile: he loves technology. And so he just instantly thought this will work.'

It was the line about working closely with the world's leading tech companies that was particularly surprising to those who had been following the app's development. Two days earlier there had been something of a bombshell announcement from Apple and Google. The two superpowers in mobile phone operating systems, who had once had a fairly amicable relationship, were these days bitter rivals, Apple boasting that its platform was far more stable and privacy-conscious, Google insisting that Android was more open and innovative. But now, in this time of crisis, the two had come together to promise help in the battle against the virus. They had noticed governments and software developers working on contact tracing so, 'in this spirit of collaboration, Google and Apple are announcing a joint effort to enable the use of Bluetooth technology to help governments and health agencies reduce the spread of the virus, with user privacy and security central to the design.' Great! – so all of those tricky problems of making Bluetooth work without draining the battery would be solved, and the NHS app could speed ahead?

Not so fast. Look at that line about user privacy. Apple and Google quickly made it clear that only certain apps would be allowed to use their software toolkits, known as APIs. The companies favoured a decentralized approach, whereby most of the data is kept on the smartphones, and the matching of contacts takes place between the phones, rather than a centralized model whereby the health authority does the matching on its computer.

So the NHS team faced a dilemma: forge ahead, battling against Bluetooth issues that would be hard to overcome without the co-operation of Apple and Google, or abandon much of the work they had done so far.

Privacy campaigners and many software engineers were adamant that it would be foolish to continue down the centralized route. Among them was Dr Michael Veale, a University College London academic specializing in digital rights. He was part of a group called DP-3T (Decentralized Privacy-Preserving Proximity Tracing), which had been working on building decentralised apps even before the announcement from Apple and Google. When DP-3T unveiled its plans on 7 April, Dr Veale made clear the consortium's view on the path the NHS was taking. 'We are opposed to data being collected centrally, as this raises questions over future intended purposes of individual information, and will affect the adoption of any such app.'

By now, the NHS team was under pressure to reveal more about its thinking on privacy, and had begun to talk to outsiders, including Michael Veale. He made clear in private that he thought they had chosen the wrong option. After the Apple/Google announcement he remembers talking to them about it. 'I said, "This doesn't work with what you're planning to do. This is obviously going to lead to Bluetooth problems down the line. Are you thinking of changing your approach because you're going to end up like Singapore?" The message came back that this did not present a problem, or prevent us "from doing sensible things with Bluetooth".

I was getting a similar message from my contacts on the app team: every time I suggested that they must be having a hard time getting it to work in the background, they insisted that their developers had come up with a clever workaround. They even suggested that they had discovered things that surprised the tech giants. A text arrived: 'Our security guys started speaking in detail with Apple/Google who are now learning from what we have done over the past few weeks and are amending their plans accordingly.' But what, I kept asking, were the benefits of a centralized app? It seemed to be all about allowing the epidemiologists to see what was going on and make decisions, rather than letting the app just trigger alerts automatically. Even though this might sound harmless, allowing anyone to see the data was going to be a no-no for the privacy campaigners.

Another message came through. 'The NHSX approach is that the contact events of a positive user, with their consent, get sent anonymously to the backend, so our epidemiologists can understand the infection pathway before cascading warnings.' But this suggested that they were still wedded to the idea of sending out alerts after a user reported symptoms, rather than waiting for a positive test, which might take time – and that meant they had to be careful about sending out too many false alarms.

It was full speed ahead with the centralized app, then, which by now was undergoing its first proper trial with servicemen and women at RAF Leeming in North Yorkshire. We were invited to film it on an embargoed basis, and as I was not allowed to venture far from my Ealing loft I had to brief a local cameraman about the shots we needed. He called me halfway through the shoot to explain how difficult an assignment it was proving. The base was following the same social-distancing rules as everywhere else, so the trial seemed to consist mainly of leaving phones running the app next to each other on a table to see what happened.

We had to wait until the following week to broadcast my report, when the Health Secretary revealed that the trial was taking place and was going well. 'The more people who sign up for this new app when it goes live, the better informed our response will be,' Matt Hancock told the House of Commons, 'and the better we can therefore protect the NHS.' And a few days later the head of NHSX, Matthew Gould, told MPs on a select committee that the app would be ready for deployment within two or three weeks.

But by then, late April, more doubts were emerging about the strategic decision to go down the centralized route rather than change tack. Other countries had wrestled with the same dilemma. Some, notably France and Australia, followed the same path as the UK, but across Europe more and more countries decided that it would be simpler to work with the Apple/Google toolkit.

Germany, perhaps the most privacy-conscious country on earth, had been clear that it favoured a centralized approach, but suddenly announced a U-turn. Michael Veale's DP-3T decentralized app group had been lobbying hard, and had found they had a perhaps surprising ally. 'The cybersecurity agency in Germany had sent really stern warnings about fundamental risks in the German centralized app that were being ignored by the health ministry.' Chancellor Merkel came down on the side of the security experts rather than the health minister.

But my sources continued to paint a picture of an NHSX project confident that it was overcoming technology problems and heading rapidly towards roll-out. They were brainstorming ideas about how to encourage downloads by promising faster release from lockdown – 'Perhaps we'll say to Sheffield, only twenty-five per cent of you have installed the app: you can't open up until you've got to fifty per cent like Newcastle,' mused one external adviser.

First, however, a much bigger trial than the one at RAF Leeming was needed. I was told this would take place on an island – though not which one – and scoured the map for inspiration. The Orkneys and Shetland were too remote and Scottish – while this was supposed to end up as an app for the whole UK, the Scottish government was casting a sceptical eye on its progress and would not guarantee its participation. Similar issues appeared to rule out Anglesey off the coast of north-west Wales, and the Isle of Man.

I concluded that the only sizeable and suitable island off the coast of England was the Isle of Wight – and I turned out to be right. During lockdown this island a few miles off the coast of Hampshire had very little traffic across the Solent from the mainland, so even if its 140,000 residents were a little older and less likely to own a smartphone than the average UK citizen, it seemed not a bad place to track transmission of the virus across a community.

The trial got under way on 5 May, with exhortations from the local council, the Isle of Wight MP Bob Seely and Matt Hancock for everyone to get involved. Indeed, the Health Secretary said the public across the country would have a 'duty' to download the app when it became available after the trial, and it would be crucial in getting 'our liberty back' as plans to ease the lockdown took shape.

I had been promised sight of the app for weeks and, although it was in theory restricted to Isle of Wight residents at this stage, I was shown how to download it. My first impression was that it was extremely simple and not very exciting – although perhaps that was the point. Once it was installed you needed to give it permission to use Bluetooth and to send you notifications, and then you were presented with a plain vanilla homepage. This featured just two things: the current government advice on stopping the spread of the virus, and a question – how are you feeling today?

If you chose the menu option 'I feel unwell', you were then asked about the only two COVID-19 symptoms recognized by the Department of Health at that time: a continuous cough or a high temperature. If, unlike me, you were an Isle of Wight resident, reporting those symptoms would lead to an instruction to self-isolate and to call an 0800 number to have a swab test delivered to your home.

What happened next, in terms of alerting the people with whom you had been in contact, was not entirely clear to me then, nor I suspect to the islanders. But no matter: the blizzard of publicity about the app did the trick. Whatever the murmurings of privacy campaigners about the lack of a proper data protection policy, islanders were soon downloading NHS COVID-19 in droves.

Eventually, over 54,000 people installed the app, to the delight of the NHSX team leaders, who were on the island nervously awaiting this first public outing of a project they genuinely believed could save lives and reduce the damage to the economy by allowing us all to emerge from lockdown. Sure, some of those people were, like me, on the mainland, but they were confident that they had reached at least half of the adult smartphone owners on the island. Bob Seely, the MP, hit back at those who had wondered whether an elderly population would embrace this new technology. 'I want to turn around in two weeks' time and challenge the rest of the United Kingdom to do as well as the Isle of Wight,' he said, reflecting the mood music from the government about a successful trial being followed by a national roll-out by the end of May.

But in retrospect that was the high point for the app. It would never be glad, confident morning again. The day after the trial started, the *Financial Times* published a story saying that the NHS had started work on a second contact tracing app, this time a decentralized one based on the Apple/Google toolkit.

'Vastly overwritten', said my NHSX contacts, trying to downplay the significance of the move while also maintaining that if a decision was made to switch it would be relatively simple, like taking an engine out of a Formula One car and installing another. But it was becoming obvious that a gulf was opening up between the app team and Number 10, Downing Street. 'The danger is that this narrative becomes self-fulfilling because it appears Downing Street is getting nervous,' said one senior figure. Another sign of the shifting sands was that the government had brought in a big hitter from the business world, the former chief executive of TalkTalk, Baroness Dido Harding, to finally get a comprehensive manual contact tracing programme under way as well as having oversight of the app. Cynics wondered whether the woman who had presided over a massive data breach at TalkTalk was really going to inspire confidence, but it was clear she had the personal backing of the Prime Minister and would henceforth be as influential in deciding the future of the project as Matt Hancock – or perhaps more.

By now I had understood that the version of the app being tested on the Isle of Wight had severe limitations, which were also becoming evident to some residents. You could use it to report symptoms and order a test, for example, but you could not enter the result of that test into the app. What I had not realized at first was that this meant the alerts being sent to contacts of people who had reported symptoms were of the mildest kind – in fact, they were identical to the 'Stay alert, control the virus, save lives' advice we were all getting at that time. And that this was never followed up with news about whether your contact had tested positive or not meant that people were left confused and in limbo.

The NHSX team insisted this was still a useful 'behavioural nudge'; that they were getting useful data from the trial. In any case, as May rolled on they were working on version 2 – the one that would be rolled out nationally as the NHS COVID-19 app. This was going to be far superior in two ways: it would include more symptoms, and it would be better integrated with the testing operation.

In fact, in a complete about-turn from version 1, alerts would not be sent out when someone reported symptoms, but only once they had received a positive test result, triggering warnings to their close contacts that they must go into quarantine for 14 days. While the Oxford scientific advisers, notably Christophe Fraser, were still adamant that early alerts triggered by reported symptoms were vital, it seemed a new realism had infected the team. If they were going to get an app out soon without undermining public confidence with lots of false alerts, a simpler message was needed.

But getting there still presented challenges. Weeks after a loss of sense of smell and taste had been acknowledged elsewhere as a symptom of coronavirus, England's chief medical officer Chris Whitty added it to the persistent cough and fever the NHS recognized as signs people might be ill. (It was another much less fancy app, the ZOE COVID Symptom Study, which had been quick to highlight the loss of sense of smell and taste. Launched in late March, it had persuaded several million people to log their symptoms daily.) Now

Professor Whitty and the three chief medical officers for Scotland, Wales and Northern Ireland got involved in framing the next version of the app, coming up with four questions for users about their health and providing a complex framework to weight the answers.

This resulted in an extraordinarily intricate flow chart which the app developers had to build into version 1 before it went live. By now, in the second half of May, the plan was for this too to be tested on the Isle of Wight before the national roll-out. When I was shown the chart by someone on the team, I told them it made my head hurt.

Apparently there was the same reaction in Downing Street. A couple of days later my phone pinged with this message: 'In confidence: PM has just over-ruled that slide from the Chief Medical Officers that made your head hurt so we now have to go back to the drawing board on a different logic . . .'

By now, a government that had been given the benefit of the doubt by most people at the beginning of the pandemic, and a Prime Minister whose own battle with the virus had won him sympathy, were under mounting pressure after a series of mis-steps, amid the growing realization that the UK was near the top of the league when it came to deaths from COVID-19. On 21 May, hoping to ease that pressure, Boris Johnson announced that England would have a 'world-beating' track-and-trace system from the beginning of June. It quickly became clear that this was a manual contact tracing programme, and Downing Street briefed that the app was likely to come along a couple of weeks later. There was still a sense on the app team that just one more push was needed to get it over the line.

But the following day a story broke which was to dominate the news agenda for the next week, and undoubtedly made Downing Street even more keen not to launch something that might not work perfectly. The *Guardian* and the *Daily Mirror* revealed that in late March, when everybody had been told to stay at home, the Prime Minister's chief adviser Dominic Cummings had travelled to Durham to stay in a cottage on his family's farm while suffering from symptoms of the coronavirus. Over the next few days, first cabinet ministers, then the Prime Minister, and then Dominic Cummings himself, appeared in front of the cameras to defend what appeared to be a flagrant breach of the government's guidelines. As more details emerged about the affair, notably Cummings' half-hour drive to Barnard Castle to test his eyesight the day before the trip home to London, many people reacted with a mixture of laughter, derision and fury. An opinion poll carried out for the Reuters Institute in the last week of May found that less than half of people surveyed trusted the government to give them accurate information about the pandemic, down from two-thirds in mid-April.

For a project that was all about persuading more than half the population to trust the government enough to put software on their phones which could in theory be used for mass surveillance, this was deeply concerning. 'Barnard Castle was a head-in-hands moment – that was when trust was lost,' a member of the app team told me months later. As May drew to a close, the Health Secretary was still promising a national roll-out in a 'couple of weeks', but by now the early enthusiasm on the Isle of Wight was fading, and people were getting restless for news. One of my contacts on the project told me the political environment was not helping – 'The Cummings scandal will do untold damage.'

In early June version 2 of the app, featuring more symptoms and the ability to report tests, was ready for trials. From around the world, however, more evidence was coming in that showed that Bluetooth was not great at measuring distance – and that applied to all apps, centralized and decentralized. Don't worry too much about this, I was told: these apps were public health tools, not scientific measuring instruments, and their accuracy should be measured against humans, who would be pretty poor at remembering how close they were to someone and for how long three days ago.

Now, this seemed a fair argument, if it weren't for the fact that the NHSX team was going through the complex process of having the app registered *as* a medical device with the Medicines and Healthcare products Regulatory Agency – just one of the bureaucratic hurdles they now complained about having to clear. While the team kept promising that big things were about to happen – 'Version 2 will roll out on the Isle of Wight on

8 June' – I could hear growing frustration in their voices about the roadblocks being placed in their path by Downing Street, which they described as 'extremely risk-averse', demanding that the app be 'bullet-proof' before it was launched.

Meanwhile, other countries were moving ahead. France launched its centralised Stop-COVID app, which had drawn heavy criticism from privacy campaigners, and digital minister Cédric O said 600,000 downloads in the first few hours was 'a good start'. Singapore, which by now seemed to have accepted that its app just was not up to the job, announced plans to give all citizens a wearable device in the hope that this would do a better job than a smartphone. On 14 June Germany became the biggest country to launch a decentralized app on the Apple/Google platform. It quickly outstripped France in terms of downloads, with something approaching 10 per cent of the population installing it within a few days.

But in the UK, ministers were repeatedly asked about the timetable for the NHSX app's roll-out, and grew more and more shy and non-committal in their answers. The business minister Nadhim Zahawi said on television programme the app would 'be running as soon as we think it is robust', and was eventually cajoled into saying that it would be out by the end of the month. Pressed at a Downing Street news conference, Matt Hancock would only say, 'when the time is right', and made it clear he wanted to focus on the manual tracing programme. Then on 17 June his junior Health Minister, Lord Bethell, gave the app a powerful kick into the long grass. 'We are seeking to get something going for the winter, but it isn't the priority for us at the moment,' he told a select committee.

That evening we learned that Matthew Gould and Geraint Lewis, the two most senior figures from NHSX running the app project, would be returning to their main jobs, and that a new man would be taking over. Simon Thompson was an executive at the online retailer Ocado who some time previously had briefly worked for Apple. The message from the NHS PR team was that this was nothing to be excited about – the plan had always been for Gould and Lewis to mastermind the development of the app and then hand it over to someone else to oversee it in operation. But we smelled a rat.

The following day, just before lunchtime, my colleague Leo Kelion, who ran the BBC's online technology news operation, rang me with an extraordinary development. A source had told him that the government was going to announce in a couple of hours that the centralized app was being ditched, and they would be switching to a decentralized model based on the Apple/Google toolkit. As there was only one source we could not go with the story yet, Leo emphasized, but we had to be ready.

But I had my own source. I texted them, 'I'm told you're going Apple/Google.'

Back came one word: 'Yep.'

That meant we could break it straight away, so Leo wrote an online story and I tweeted this: 'BBC scoop – NHS abandons centralized contact tracing app, moves to Apple/Google decentralized model.'

Within minutes I was breaking the story live on the BBC News Channel, and when I returned to my computer I found a Twitter Direct Message from what I think is known as a 'very senior source' wanting to brief me on background about the decision.

As the afternoon wore on, details emerged first in private, and then in public at the Downing Street press conference with Matt Hancock and Dido Harding, about what had gone wrong with the app project. That Isle of Wight trial that had been such a success? Actually it had been a bit of a disaster – Baroness Harding revealed that while the app had been good at detecting Android phones, it was no good at spotting Apple devices. In fact, it only detected 4 per cent of nearby iPhones. We also learned for the first time that a decentralized app, developed by the London branch of the Swiss firm Zühlke, had also been trialled. It had proved much better at spotting iPhones, but surprisingly less effective than the original version at using Bluetooth to measure the distance between two phones.

At that Downing Street briefing Baroness Harding made clear her scepticism about the effectiveness of either type of app. 'What we've done in really rigorously testing both our own COVID-19 app and the Google/Apple version is demonstrate that none of them are working sufficiently well enough to be actually reliable to determine whether any of us should self-isolate for two weeks, [and] that's true across the world.' Standing alongside her – or rather 2 metres apart – the Health Secretary struck a similar downbeat note about any kind of app being rolled out soon, while also suggesting that a lack of co-operation from Apple had stymied the project.

If Matt Hancock had hoped to deflect some of the blame it did not work. Apple was furious, and also insisted that it had not, as was claimed, been briefed about the switch to a decentralized app. And the next day the front pages of the newspapers were brutal – especially those which were normally sympathetic to the government. The failure of the app left the government's contact tracing strategy 'in disarray', said *The Times*. For the *Daily Telegraph*, which dubbed Matt Hancock 'hapless and app-less', the project was a 'national embarrassment'. Worst of all, the conservative *Daily Mail*, the most powerful paper in Britain, asked 'How Many More Corona Fiascos?', detailing a string of U-turns on everything from testing to the availability of protective equipment, and laying most of the blame at Hancock's door.

It did not get much better over the coming days when, at Prime Minister's Questions, Boris Johnson claimed that no country in the world had a working contact tracing app. Challenged by the Prime Minister to name a country with a functioning app, the Labour leader Keir Starmer fired back: 'Germany'. Beaten again by the Germans: much of the press and social media treated the affair as though it was another humiliation akin to repeated defeats in penalty shoot-outs.

For those from the private sector who had got involved in the app it was further confirmation that governments are just no good at managing IT projects. That included the tech luminary who had first contacted me about it back in March. Another message from them pinged on my phone: 'I'm sorry to have wasted your time. I had no idea, not even the slightest sensation, that this would be the outcome.' I rang to say no need to apologize – it had been a great story – and got an outpouring of frustration about the nightmare of pushing out an app amidst public and regulatory scrutiny and political infighting, compared with the 'just do it' experience of launching it in the private sector.

So who was to blame – and was it quite the catastrophic failure it seemed? It struck me that much of the reaction, particularly on social media, was a bit unfair. Every time I tweeted about the story, a host of people claimed it had gone wrong because it was all about a twisted plan by Dominic Cummings to give contracts to his mates in various companies and then grab everyone's data.

For the record, the Cummings affair, when he appeared to have broken at least the spirit of lockdown rules, did nothing to improve the morale of the people working on the app – but he had absolutely no connection with VMware Pivotal or Zühlke, the two main contractors working on the app, and indeed appeared to have shown little interest in the whole project.

Neither was it clear that it was a massive technology failure. The team tasked with building a centralized app had to battle against the vagaries of Bluetooth with little or no co-operation from Apple, and in the circumstances did a pretty good job. And a few days after the Downing Street press briefing, I discovered that Baroness Harding had mistakenly exaggerated the failings of the app during the Isle of Wight trial.

I wrote a long piece about the whole affair, quoting her line about only 4 per cent of iPhones being detected. A technology expert I knew who lived on the island wrote to me to say the piece was good except for a key mistake: 'That 4 per cent is only when the app is asleep in the background, after some tens of minutes of non-use by either phone. Which is just a small percentage of the total iPhone-to-iPhone interactions.' I put him right, reading from a transcript of the briefing. But he then revealed he had been at a briefing given by the chief technology officer of NHSX to people on the island – and it was clear that his figures were the right ones. It seemed that once Baroness Harding had briefed out the wrong figure, apparently based on misunderstanding a document, nobody else felt able to correct her. A few weeks later, a paper by scientists at the Alan

Turing Institute, who had been involved in the project, appeared to show they had made some progress in making Bluetooth more accurate as a means of measuring the distance between two phones. This was research that would help improve both centralized and decentralized apps.

And while Boris Johnson's line that no country in the world had developed a functioning contact tracing app was overstated, there were reasons to ask whether anyone had really cracked this problem yet. Sure, by mid-July more than 15 million Germans had downloaded the Corona-Warn app, but there was no news on how many people had been alerted to contacts with an infected person and sent into quarantine. What was more concerning were the replies we got when we asked both Germany and Switzerland, which had pioneered the decentralized approach using the Apple/Google toolkit, whether there would be some data soon on their apps' effectiveness. According to Germany's Robert Koch Institute, which was managing its app, the decentralized approach mandated by the tech giants meant they would not have access to information about how many people had been alerted to go into quarantine, or how many false alarms had been sent out. The log history it would need to tap into to learn the answers 'remains with the users, encrypted on their smartphones'. The Swiss health department also ascribed its lack of data about its app's effectiveness to the Apple/Google model: 'We hence have the same limitations in terms of statistics. We don't know – and have no way of finding out – the number of people warned by the app or any false positives/false negatives.'

Privacy campaigners who had urged the UK to follow Germany's lead and switch to using the Apple/Google toolkit felt vindicated by the government's belated U-turn. But a few people in the technology world were dismayed that the two tech giants seemed to be deciding for governments where the balance should be struck between preserving privacy and fighting the pandemic. Tom Loosemore, who had been co-founder of the Government Digital Service, which brought a somewhat more nimble approach to public sector IT, called what Apple and Google had done a troubling display of unaccountable power. They had made, he argued, 'a huge, global, public health policy decision – a decision that I believe should be the preserve of elected governments. They alone had determined where the balance between privacy and public health should lie.'

As the development of apps based on the Apple/Google API continued around the world in 2020, it was to become clear that their solution was far from perfect. Apple, for instance, limited the amount of data apps could extract to judge the distance between two phones, making readings quite inaccurate. Although an update did eventually improve matters, countries found themselves beholden to these Californian behemoths at the very same time that they were talking of regulating them more strictly.

Of course, Bluetooth contact tracing apps approved by Google and Apple were not the only option. It was notable that the only countries where technology did appear to play a significant and successful role in controlling the spread of the virus were those like South Korea, Taiwan and China, where privacy concerns were largely brushed aside.

In the end, though, the UK's app fiasco was born out of the exaggerated faith of politicians in the power of technology. When the project was born in early March the ramshackle manual contact tracing programme was rapidly being overwhelmed by thousands of cases, and an app seemed a magical solution to a government confident that Britain was a world leader in everything from artificial intelligence to quantum computing. By contrast, Germany had an extensive regionally-based, old-fashioned test-and-trace system which was key to its relative success in controlling the virus, so for its government an app was nice to have but not essential. That in turn meant it did not have to be perfect at launch, just good enough to supplement the work of an army of manual contact tracers.

The technology of the smartphone social era was proving useful if not transformational in this healthcare crisis. But the billions of mobile computers in people's pockets and the networks that connected them were proving extremely effective at one thing: spreading misinformation about the virus and what was behind it.

13

Fake News, 5G and the Virus

This book has been about the conflicting emotions we have felt during an era when technology became more personal. The hope was that it would liberate us, make us wealthier and happier; the fear was that it would endanger our children, undermine our democracy and make giant unaccountable technology companies even more powerful. During the coronavirus crisis, we experienced the best and the worst of what smartphones and social media could do for us. As we have seen, they helped us keep in touch with loved ones and colleagues while forced to stay at home – indeed, many discovered that they could be more productive working at their kitchen table than catching a crowded train to an office building in some city centre. They also helped, in a modest way, the scientists and policymakers looking for a way out of the crisis.

But in the debit column a phenomenon that was already present, misinformation spread by social media, became much more evident and much more dangerous. A tidal wave of lies and hoaxes, rumours and scams swept around the world, spread on WhatsApp and Facebook, Snapchat, Twitter and TikTok. A population hungry for information about the coronavirus had a vast number of sources of news that would not have been available if the pandemic had happened before the social smartphone era, but too often they were not reliable.

Among the stories being shared in February 2020 was the idea that coronavirus had been engineered in a lab – either by China or the

United States, depending on your politics. Or perhaps its dangers had been exaggerated – it was little more than a mild form of flu. There were dodgy cures and tips: drink more hot water; try not to drink ice; if you can hold your breath for ten seconds and not cough, then you definitely don't have the virus. These ideas often arrived on phones labelled as coming from 'my friend who knows a nurse working in ICU' or 'a doctor friend who has been talking to colleagues in Northern Italy'. Later, of course, tips such as drinking bleach or taking a new 'wonder drug', hydroxychloroquine, came not from fictitious strangers but from world leaders such as Donald Trump or Brazil's Jair Bolsonaro.

Then there was the theory that one of the world's biggest philanthropists, a tech billionaire who was spending much of his fortune on trying to improve global health, was up to no good when it came to the coronavirus. Bill Gates, the story went, had a devilish plan to use vaccines as a cover to insert microchips under people's skin and then control their minds. A TED talk back in 2015 where the Microsoft founder warned, 'If anything kills over ten million people over the next few decades, it is likely to be a highly infectious virus rather than war,' was somehow seen as evidence of malevolent intent rather than prescience.

At first this all might have seemed harmless enough – after all, people have always believed weird and wonderful things about illnesses and how they should be treated. But in an era that saw millions rely for their primary news source on Facebook or WhatsApp, the World Health Organization warned that we were in the middle of an 'infodemic' that could cause huge damage, perhaps making it less likely that people would trust that a vaccine was safe when one came along.

In late February 2020 an epidemiologist from the University of East Anglia, Paul Hunter, told my *Tech Tent* programme about the lessons learned from the Ebola virus in West Africa in 2016. Very similar rumours to those around the coronavirus had spread: that it was all a hoax, that it was a money-making exercise, that wearing masks and other protective equipment was just an overreaction.

'People who believed conspiracy theories about Ebola were less likely to adopt safe practices, especially safe funeral practices. And so they were putting themselves at an increased risk of getting the infection and ultimately increased risk of dying.'

But by the time of the coronavirus pandemic there was one new conspiracy theory that was more deluded, yet apparently also more widespread, than any other – and it concerned the very technology that was going to make spreading information around the world via smartphones even easier and faster: 5G, it alleged, was behind the coronavirus. It turned out that in Wuhan, where COVID-19 originated, a huge array of 5G masts had been turned on just a few weeks earlier – or at least that was the claim.

From this original lightbulb going off in someone's head, multiple stories about the links between 5G and the virus took off. When hundreds of passengers on cruise ships came down with COVID-19 it was obviously caused by their brand-new communications systems, which must have featured 5G. Then there was the idea that actually the coronavirus was nothing more serious than the common cold, and what 5G did was weaken the immune system so that the body could not deal with it. And it was no good pointing out that the virus was spreading in countries like Iran where 5G had not been rolled out. 'That's what you think,' said one of the more extreme conspiracy-mongers, adamant that 5G was being developed as a secret weapon around the world.

As well as some of social media's more exotic characters, the 5G virus theory was also being pushed by celebrities, among them one of Britain's best-known television hosts. In an exchange with the ITV *Good Morning* programme's consumer editor Alice Beer, who described the theory as 'not true' and 'incredibly stupid', Eamonn Holmes had this to say: 'What I don't accept is mainstream media immediately slapping that down as not true when they don't know it's not true. It's very easy to say it is not true because it suits the state narrative.'

Leaving aside the attack on the mainstream media by a man whose entire career was about being mainstream, this was an extraordinary attack on science at a dangerous time, when it was vital that the public should be given reliable information about the virus. The presenter did make an apology the following day, and the media regulator Ofcom issued what it described as 'guidance' to ITV, calling his remarks 'ambiguous' and 'ill-judged', and warning they 'risked undermining viewers' trust in advice from public authorities and scientific evidence'.

But the damage had been done. More wild rumours spread: the Thursday-night 'Clap for Carers' ritual, when people came out onto their streets to applaud NHS workers, was apparently a conspiracy to cover up the noise of 5G cables being laid. The Nightingale hospitals being rapidly constructed in places like London's Excel Centre to accommodate coronavirus patients were actually giant morgues, ready for when the network was switched on.

Again, all of this might sound bonkers but insignificant, but it was having an effect in the real world on people doing vital work. The first hint of what was going on came in a video shared widely on Facebook and Twitter. A woman, out of shot and presumably holding a phone, approaches a couple of telecoms engineers working in the street, laying fibre-optic cables. She asks them what they are doing, suggesting that they are breaking the law because they are not key workers (even though what they are doing has been classified as essential work). Then she tells them the world may already be facing the first case of a 'viral or bacterial mutation' due to the 5G roll-out, and presents her conspiracy theory: 'You know when they turn this on, it's going to kill everyone, and that's why they're building the hospitals,' she explains. 'Do you have children? Do you have parents? When they turn that switch on, bye-bye Momma. Are they paying you well enough to kill people?'

The engineers are remarkably patient, smiling and saying they can refer her to their boss. But across the UK there were far more serious incidents. Over the next three months around 90 mobile phone masts were set on fire by people apparently convinced that 5G was a threat to life and limb – even though most of the sites they attacked were actually part of the 4G network.

As telecoms executives pointed out, the real danger to life and limb was in damaging vital communications infrastructure, which in some cases involved networks used by the emergency services during a pandemic.

Tracking down the first mention of a link between 5G and the coronavirus is not easy. A fact-checking site called Newsguard reckoned that the first sighting was as early as 20 January, on a French conspiracy site, Les Moutons Enragés. It asked, using the same terminology as the woman in the video, 'Could we already be facing the first case of "a viral or bacterial mutation" due to the roll-out of 5G?' The answer of course was no, but a couple of days later a Belgian newspaper carried an interview with a doctor who claimed the virus outbreak could be linked to 5G masts installed near Wuhan in 2019. That piece was quickly taken down but, just like a virus released into the wild, it had already spread to that wonderful invention, social media – and from there into the minds of millions of credulous people.

But the idea that 5G and the coronavirus were linked would not have been so potent had there not already been a substantial number of people who distrusted all of the technology of the mobile phone era. The previous spring, as the mobile networks in the UK began to announce their roll-out plans, I noticed a mushrooming of anti-5G groups. Search for the term 5G on Facebook and you would find that just about every local area had a group dedicated to stopping its roll out on health grounds. Twitter and Instagram were also fertile areas for those spreading the message that the technology was not safe.

They came armed with all sorts of facts and figures and research documents. Many quoted from a letter apparently signed by 180 scientists and doctors calling for a moratorium across Europe on the roll-out of 5G. The signatories' main concern appeared to be that 5G was a step-change in mobile communications, with the use of more masts and higher frequencies. 'The wireless telecom industry intend to outfit nearly every lamp post or utility post around the countries [sic]', they warned, 'with these wireless small-cell antennas beaming hazardous radiation next to, or into our homes, schools, working places and everywhere, 24/7.'

It sounded alarming – until you asked yourself what this 'hazardous radiation' was. The new networks might use higher-frequency waves than 2G, 3G or 4G, but that did not make them dangerous. The wireless spectrum in question was still way down in the non-ionizing part of the electromagnetic spectrum, which meant, according to the physicist and cancer researcher David Robert Grimes in a BBC Reality Check article, that 'it lacks sufficient energy to break apart DNA and cause cellular damage.' It was ionizing *radiation* – X-rays and ultraviolet light – which could do that.

As a non-scientist I turned frequently to Dr Grimes to try to understand the issues around 5G. I had noticed him the previous year, when the *Observer* newspaper had published an article appearing to show that telecoms companies had suppressed information about links between mobile phones and cancer. The following week they had given him space to dismantle what he described as a piece 'strewn with rudimentary errors and dubious inferences'.

In particular, he zeroed in on the authors' reference to one study which appeared to show that rats exposed to intense radio frequency had higher rates of brain cancer than a control group. He pointed to all sorts of problems with the research: it turned out that the rats exposed to the radiation had lived much longer than the control group, and were therefore more likely to get cancer in old age. And in any case, no conclusions could be drawn from one study – science was about finding consistent trends across the whole body of research, and that showed no link between phone use and cancer.

But scientists like David Robert Grimes would find that challenging the views of people convinced that mobile phone networks would do them harm can become a full-time job, with no guarantee that you will have much success. Concern about the effects of electromagnetic radiation had begun long before 5G, and many people had been campaigning for years against everything from mobile phone masts to Wi-Fi networks. Those who believed the technology was harmful would come armed with research they had uncovered on the internet and quote 'respected scientists' and 'peer-reviewed articles' that backed up their case. Look more closely, and you would find that the peer-reviewed articles were in obscure journals whose business model depended on people who paid to be published, and most of the scientists were not in fields where expertise in the physics of electromagnetic radiation was a requirement.

Take that letter to the EU calling for a 5G moratorium. One of those who signed the letter was Arthur Firstenberg, an American with a degree in mathematics who had been arguing since 1996 that wireless technology was dangerous, going so far as to file a lawsuit against his neighbour, seeking damages because she refused to turn off her mobile phone. The signatories from the UK included people with doctorates in social economics and clinical psychology. There was a clutch of medical practitioners, including Dr Andrew Tresidder, a former GP who now offered flower remedies and emotional healing. Then there was Alasdair Philips, a man who described himself as a professional engineer for Powerwatch, a group that had been campaigning for 20 years against what it saw as the damaging effects of power lines, Wi-Fi, mobile phones and masts.

Over those two decades, during which the use of mobile phones and wireless technology became ubiquitous, mainstream scientists had found little or no evidence of the health impacts described by campaigners. Professor Will Stewart, president of the UK's Institution of Engineering and Technology (IET), smiled wryly when I asked him about the studies quoted by those who insisted there was such evidence. He explained how this worked:

> If you take enough variables on your parameters, you can find something that fits. If your policy is to change things until you get a positive result, you will eventually get a positive result. You won't be able to repeat it, but you will get it once, and often that's enough to start these conspiracy theories.

He said the panic around 5G had focused on the idea that the new networks would use higher frequencies and require many more masts – those 'small antennas on every lamp post' mentioned in the scary letter to the EU. But he explained more masts were only needed because of the short range of those higher frequencies, and they would each be using much less power. All the infrastructure for 5G had to conform to global safety standards set by ICNIRP, the International Commission on Non-Ionizing Radiation Protection, and tests by the telecoms regulator Ofcom on some of the first masts installed found they were well within those limits – in fact, the highest radiation reading was 0.039 per cent of the recommended exposure limit.

In a leaflet explaining all this, the IET said it had 'investigated the specific claim that 5G poses uniquely greater exposure risks to health, and our findings are emphatically "No", it does not.' But this document was published in the summer of 2020, by which time 5G concerns had spread far and wide, everywhere from the environmental movement to the wildest extremes of conspiratorial thinking, for which 5G was all part of a plan by dark forces to commit genocide. As Will Stewart from the IET acknowledged, the scientists and the telecoms industry had been far too complacent about getting their message out.

He understood why spreading conspiracy theories was appealing: 'You want something that's exciting to tell your friends. To be that, it's got to be startling, unusual, preposterous.' It was perhaps not surprising that in the era of social media, with trust in institutions in decline, people leaped to ill-informed conclusions about a technology that was essential to the way they communicated.

But it is too easy to blame social media. Just as the myth that the MMR vaccine was linked to autism had been heavily promoted by newspapers, both tabloid and broadsheet, and even by the BBC, so bad science about wireless technology got a hearing on mainstream media. Back in 2007, the venerable BBC current affairs flagship *Panorama* broadcast an edition with the title 'Wi-Fi: A Warning Signal'. To dramatic, doom-laden music it explored the move to install Wi-Fi in schools, suggesting this posed a real danger to children's health because they were being subjected to the same sort of radiation as came from mobile phone masts. The programme toured Norwich, and found worrying signs that Wi-Fi networks were springing up everywhere across the city and its schools. One key witness who was shown carrying out tests of radiation from masts and Wi-Fi routers was the aforementioned Alasdair Philips of Powerwatch, later one of the signatories of that 5G letter to the EU. The lobby group was described as raising awareness of 'electrosmog', an emotive term which mainstream scientists do not recognize as meaningful. The programme went on to feature a woman who said she was so sensitive to radiation from a nearby mast that she had bought a tinfoil canopy to cover her bed as protection. One scientist was interviewed who insisted that there was not enough evidence to prove a threat to health – but his evidence was deemed 'controversial' because he had previously worked for the phone industry.

A few months after the broadcast the BBC Editorial Complaints Unit criticized the programme for a lack of balance. But the damage was done. At the time a group of scientists were looking into conditions such as the electrosensitivity from which the woman in the programme said she suffered, but for which there appeared to be no physiological explanation. The scientists conducted a study which indicated that people who said they were sensitive to electromagnetic radiation could not tell whether a Wi-Fi router was switched on or off.

Then one of the scientists, a German clinical psychologist, Professor Michael Witthöft, wondered whether what he described as 'sensationalist media reports' were having an effect on these people, and decided to stage another experiment. He gathered together a group of electrosensitive people and played them a section of the *Panorama* film. Then he told the group they were going to be subjected to radiation, strapping an antenna to their heads with a cable leading to a Wi-Fi router with a blinking light. The router was not actually emitting anything and the antennae were fake, but they were told it was all going to be switched on for a quarter of an hour. In 2020, Professor Witthöft told the BBC Radio programme *File on 4* what happened next: 'We were quite surprised, because two of our participants told us during those fifteen minutes, "Please switch off the signal, because my headache is becoming too strong."'

The results of one small experiment should not be overplayed, but this was one of a number of studies which appeared to show the existence of what is called a 'nocebo' effect. Just as being given a placebo – a dummy pill – can make you feel better, if you are told, say, that even holding a phone to your head could be harmful, you may develop a headache.

By the time 5G began to be talked about, there had been plenty more reports like the *Panorama* programme raising the idea that sensitivity to electromagnetic radiation was a serious health issue. Very few people were still calling for Wi-Fi to be banned from schools, but there were any number of groups campaigning against mobile phone masts, and warning that 'electrosmog' was causing untold misery. There was also a thriving little industry making products to protect people from the harmful effects of electromagnetic radiation. On a site called EMF Protection you could get a protective canopy for your bed for as little as £939 – although if you wanted the deluxe version for a four-poster you would have to pay upwards of £1,600. There were radiation monitors, protective hoodies for £169, leggings for £112, and even a baseball cap – literally a tinfoil hat – for just £29.99. The site featured endorsements from happy customers: 'My wife and I wore these on our recent transatlantic flights that featured Wi-Fi and active phone links,' wrote one, 'and it was the smoothest, least headachy flight ever.'

Hardly surprising, then, that everything from vague health concerns to wild-eyed conspiracy theories about 5G spread rapidly. Among the most fertile areas for campaigns against the new networks was south-west England. In 2019, the town council in Totnes in Devon said it would oppose 5G until councillors were confident that it was safe. Frome Town Council in Somerset said it would not endorse the roll-out 'until there is more independent scientific consensus that 5G wireless radiation is harmless to humans and the environment'. But it was Glastonbury, the supposed site of the tomb of King Arthur and home to every kind of mystic, soothsayer and alternative therapist, that was the epicentre of opposition to 5G.

In 2019 the Glastonbury Festival, which is actually based 7 miles away in the village of Pilton, had taken place just a few weeks after

EE launched the UK's first 5G network. The mobile company had decided that here was a chance to show off the technology – after all, one of the main advantages of 5G was that it would bring far greater capacity to a network and, with 200,000 people all using their mobile phones at the same time, the festival had long been one massive 'notspot'.

But naturally there was fierce opposition. A petition accused the organizers and EE of using festivalgoers as guinea pigs, calling 5G 'a "weapons-grade" phone technology that has sparked health concerns and been linked with a spate of suicides at Bristol University'. The trial went ahead – although as hardly anyone at the festival besides a few journalists had a 5G handset it was hard to know what it proved. Nevertheless, the Electrosensitivity UK group insisted that site workers had reported 'bad headaches, nosebleeds and digestive issues'. (Frequent festivalgoers might think this sounds like the usual Glastonbury hangover.)

By now Glastonbury Town Council, which was run by the Green Party, had passed a motion opposing the roll-out of 5G in the area, 'based on the precautionary principle, until further information is revealed from a newly convened 5G advisory committee.' And while there were plenty of people in the town instinctively suspicious of the technology, the council had also been vigorously lobbied by visiting campaigners, notably one Christopher Baker. Described by the Electro-Sensitivity UK newsletter as an EMF consultant, he told councillors that Glastonbury could take a lead in blocking 5G that others would follow. Mr Baker was then appointed as a member of that 5G advisory committee, which was to take a deep dive into the technology and advise the council on whether it was safe.

This committee had a somewhat grand and ambitious mission for a town council – which had, after all, little or no say in planning decisions around the siting of mobile phone masts. Yet it was asked by councillors to advise them 'on the safety or otherwise of 5G cellular network technology', and on whether or not they should continue to oppose the roll-out of 5G. Its members were instructed to 'approach experts to give presentations and specialist advice to the committee on the safety or otherwise of 5G cellular network technology' and 'collect evidence demonstrating the safety or otherwise of 5G cellular network technology from robust sources'.

In a way you could see this as admirable. Glastonbury was showing the UK and the rest of the world that you needed to look at all of the scientific evidence before coming to a conclusion about something as important as a revolutionary new technology. After being convened in July and holding 13 meetings through the autumn and winter, the committee delivered its report in April 2020 at the height of the UK's coronavirus lockdown – and at a time when theories about a link between the virus and 5G were spreading rapidly. In his foreword, the committee's chairman, Green Party councillor Jon Cousins, made it clear that this report was likely to have an impact far beyond the local area. 'Glastonbury', he wrote, 'has been described as "*a town that punches above its weight*", influencing other councils and levels of government both locally and nationally.'

The report came down firmly on the side of those who thought 5G unsafe. It said the council should call for MPs to hold an inquiry into the technology, and demand that the government undertake an independent scientific study into the non-thermal effects of 5G and electromagnetic hypersensitivity. On top of that, Glastonbury Council needed to lobby ICNIRP – the International Commission on Non-Ionizing Radiation Protection – to change the way it set guidelines for emissions from phone masts. The global body needed to look at 'the non-thermal effects of radiofrequency EMFs' – in other words, the unproven claims that everything from Wi-Fi to 2G, 3G and 4G can cause damage to the human body.

Even if the UK parliament and the international standards body were unlikely to leap into action at the behest of one Somerset council, the report seemed like a serious contribution to the debate about 5G. After all, the committee of nine councillors and nine external members had consulted leading scientists and had combed through all of the research – hadn't they?

A few weeks after the report was published I was contacted by one of those external members, who painted a very different picture of the nature of the report. Far from being a rigorous study of the science, Mark Swann told me, it had been hijacked by conspiracy theorists.

Mr Swann, who had a degree in physics, had responded to an advert in the local paper calling for people with relevant experience to help decide whether 5G was safe. 'I joined the working group in good faith, expecting to take part in a sensible discussion about 5G,' he told me. 'Sadly the whole thing turned out to be a clueless pantomime, driven by conspiracy-theorists and sceptics.'

The nine councillors on the committee all appeared to have started with a sceptical attitude towards the technology, and had not changed their minds. But what about the nine external members? Besides Mark Swann, two others had a scientific background. Derek Cooper was a retired electronics engineer who had worked in the aerospace and defence industries, while Carol Roberts was a molecular biologist employed in the pharmaceuticals industry. All three ended up resigning before the report was published, as did another external member, David Swain, a businessman and Conservative councillor in a neighbouring town. I got in touch with Derek Cooper and David Swain and, while Carol Roberts did not want to go on the record, I got hold of her resignation letter, which made clear her dismay about how the committee had been run.

Derek Cooper told me it did not take long for him to see how the report was likely to turn out. 'I worked out that there were only four of us who were neutral. And the others were all absolutely against 5G, either strongly or weakly.' David Swain said he had joined with some experience of local politics in Glastonbury, knowing that 'quirky' views were common on the council and hoping to provide some balance:

> But even from our first meeting, it was clear that there were a handful of people there who, it didn't matter what evidence was put in front of them, they were convinced that 5G was slowly killing them, and the government was trying to roll it out to control the masses.

In his letter of resignation he wrote, 'Genuine scientific expertise has been scorned in favour of conspiracy and hearsay.'

So who were the five other members of the public invited to join the committee and lend their expertise to its deliberations? Sandra Spearing was the administrator of a group called Glastonbury Stop 5G and Smart Meters. Roy Procter, a dowser and spiritual healer, was on the board of the Chalice Well Trust, which oversees the site where, according to some Christians, Joseph of Arimathea placed the chalice that caught drops of Christ's blood during the crucifixion. Toby Hall was a believer in alternative therapies and was concerned about the impact of electromagnetic radiation, using a substance called shungite to shield his home from its effects. Susan Jones was a firm opponent of 5G, stating in the final report, 'I would recommend fibre-cable broadband as an alternative! If the government can finance 5G in my opinion they can finance fibre-cable broadband, as Labour's Jeremy Corbyn intended, had he won the election.' (The government did not 'finance' 5G – indeed, it hoped to make some money, by auctioning the necessary spectrum to the mobile networks.)

And then there was Christopher Baker, the man who had lobbied the council to take a stand on 5G in the first place. He had spent many months campaigning across the South-West against the technology, but at one stage he appeared disgruntled at the lack of support he was getting in Glastonbury. In a Facebook post in May 2019, he told local people to jolly well shape up: 'The only thing that is missing is the support from the community! I can't do this for you on my own, this is about you and for you.'

But by July he appeared to have cheered up. In a YouTube video posted that month by another anti-5G activist, John Kitson, Baker described the tactics he used to engage with Glastonbury Town Council to get the investigation under way, advising others to spend time cultivating councillors. He also appeared in videos alongside other anti-5G conspiracy theorists including Mark Steele, a man whose activities became ever more extreme during the coronavirus pandemic. I had first come across Steele and his brother Graham, who ran a company marketing motorcycle helmets with heads-up displays, some years before. Graham sent me emails, copying in the Prime Minister's office and assorted others, warning that D Notices were being issued to suppress news about microwave radiation and its impact on human health. When he started comparing the 5G roll-out to the Holocaust, which I found deeply offensive, I blocked him. Meanwhile Mark Steele was mounting a campaign of harassment against his local council in Gateshead, which he accused of installing 5G in lamp posts as part of an evil global plan to commit genocide. Then, during the lockdown, he posted videos of himself harassing telecoms engineers and warning them that they were engaged in criminal activities.

When I managed to contact Christopher Baker, he was keen to play down any connection with Mark Steele or other conspiracy theorists, insisting that he was not even an anti-5G campaigner. 'I'm more an adviser . . . All I was doing was helping to set up a process to put a formal and a robust process in place to discuss the prospects of 5G.'

But it was his presence on the committee that led to the resignation of Derek Cooper, the retired electronics engineer. Mr Cooper said the committee was supposed to be made up of people who lived in the area or had a business there, complaining that Christopher Baker did not meet that requirement because he lived in Hampshire. After the complaint was ignored, he resigned, describing Mr Baker as a 'semi-professional anti-5G activist' and pointing to a video in which Mr Baker had admitted that some of his fuel costs were paid by a benefactor.

Mr Baker told me it was true that he lived in Hampshire, but said he had long-term connections to Glastonbury, and in any case other members of the committee were from outside the town. He admitted that he did receive some funding from a benefactor, whom he refused to name. 'I don't have a lot of money, and if I travel halfway up the country to give a presentation, the least I expect is someone to contribute something towards my fuel bill.'

But if anyone played a major role in shaping the way the report turned out it was Christopher Baker. He was instrumental in choosing a number of the witnesses, and gave his own presentation in which he attacked the credibility of ICNIRP, the standards body which the committee had recommended should be lobbied to change its methods. The majority of the evidence the committee heard was from witnesses who had stated their support for a moratorium on the roll-out of 5G. They included a number of scientists who had been regulars on the anti-EMF circuit for years. Retired American professor Martin Pall gave a presentation by video link explaining how electromagnetic waves led to the production of excess calcium cells. The final report says one of the external members who later resigned maintained the argument was based on a faulty understanding of the science, and 'this unfortunately makes his whole hypothesis nonsense from the outset.' A few months earlier Professor Pall had told a conference in Germany that wireless networks would make all human beings sterile if they were not switched off within two years, and within five to seven years normal functioning of the human brain would cease.

Another scientist who gave evidence via video and backed up some of Professor Pall's claims was Professor Tom Butler, from University College, Cork. But as his specialism was business information systems, those on the committee with a background in physics and electronics refused to be impressed. There was also evidence in person from Dr Andrew Tresidder, the emotional-healing specialist who was among the collection of scientists calling for a European moratorium on 5G. His presentation focused on people claiming to suffer from 'electromagnetic stress', which he said was often not taken seriously by mainstream doctors. And some of the external members also presented their views, including Roy Procter, the spiritual healer who claims dowsing can heal 'sick houses'. In the final report, he speculated about a link between the coronavirus and 5G and recommended that the council eliminate all Wi-Fi connections.

There was one presentation from an external body wholly in favour of 5G. Hamish MacLeod and Gareth Elliott from Mobile UK, the mobile phone industry trade body, came to Glastonbury Town Hall and showed a PowerPoint presentation. They met with a somewhat hostile reception – one committee member later deriding the presentation as 'glossy', others suggesting that their questions were ignored. When I spoke to Gareth Elliott he laughed at the suggestion that a few slides amounted to something glossy, and strongly denied they had been evasive: 'We answered everything that was asked of us.' He did stress, however, that it was a cordial meeting.

But Elliott did pass on an anecdote which gave a flavour of the proceedings. One committee member, a councillor, arrived late and said that, while she was hyper-sensitive to emissions, she deemed the meeting room safe. 'It was then noted that a Wi-Fi router was operating and was in the room,' said the Mobile UK representative drily.

The chair of the committee, Councillor Jon Cousins, was insistent that allegations that the report had been hijacked by conspiracy theorists and pseudo-science were completely unfair. 'Equal weight was given to all contributions,' he said. One of the dissident committee members, Mark Swann, said the final report did not reflect that: while he counted 35 mentions of Martin Pall, whom he described as a well-known conspiracy theorist, he found no mention of radiobiology, the branch of science covering the effects of radiation on the human body.

But the word 'coronavirus' does appear several times in the report, as does Wuhan, where the pandemic began, and a couple of the committee members make explicit references to a link between the virus and 5G. Coming at a time when such conspiracy theories were rife, and were promoted in a protest march in the town by Piers Corbyn, brother of the then Labour leader, this led some of the former committee members to be worried about the reputation of Glastonbury. Councillor Cousins insisted that the Council had never suggested a link between 5G and the coronavirus. The man who had seen the report as showing that Glastonbury punched above its weight was not having it when I suggested that it had damaged the reputation of the town. I wrote a lengthy article about the affair for the BBC, which was picked up far and wide, but the document remained on the Town Council's website.

A few weeks later, however, my attention was drawn to something interesting in one of the report's appendices. One of the external members, Toby Hall, had given his own reflections on the inquiry. He asked why, when peer-reviewed science showed 5G was unsafe, were governments and regulators letting it be rolled out? His answer: 'Money, power, surveillance, and control.'

But he also had a couple of recommendations of products that would help protect against the dangers of electromagnetic radiation. One was a mineral called shungite, 'a cheap and helpful preventive, available in several Glastonbury shops'. Another was a product called the 5G Bioshield: 'We use this device and find it helpful.' Mr Hall provided a useful link to the website. It featured pictures of homes and people safely shielded within a bubble apparently generated by this helpful device. The 5G Bioshield was described as a USB key which 'provides protection for your home and family, thanks to the wearable holographic nano-layer catalyser, which can be worn or placed near to a smartphone or any other electrical, radiation or EMF-emitting device'. It went on to explain that 'through a process of quantum oscillation the 5G BioShield USB Key balances and reharmonizes the disturbing frequencies arising from the electric fog induced by devices such as laptops, cordless phones, Wi-Fi, tablets, etc.'

Already dizzy from all of this quantum oscillation, I clicked through to the checkout and found that, understandably, these miraculous devices did not come cheap. One USB key cost £339.60 including VAT, though there was a special offer that enabled you to get three for just £958.80. So what exactly was the technology behind this apparently simple device? Well, Ken Munro, whose company Pen Test Partners specialized in taking apart electronic devices to spot any security vulnerabilities, had decided on his own initiative to take a closer look. He splashed out nearly £1,000 on a three-pack so he could do a proper job.

At first sight it seemed that the USB key was in fact . . . a USB key, and, with storage of just 128MB, one of the cheapest on the market. 'So what's different,' he asked in a Pen Test Partners blogpost, 'between it and a virtually identical "crystal" USB key available from various suppliers in Shenzhen, China for around £5 per key?'

The answer, he said, appeared to be a circular sticker. 'Now, we're not 5G quantum experts, but said sticker looks remarkably like one available in sheets from stationery suppliers for less than a penny each.'

But Ken did not stop there. He proceeded to dismantle the USB key to find out if there were any whizzbang electronics inside. All he found was an LED light on the circuit board similar to those on any other USB stick made in Shenzhen. Again keen to insist that he was no expert on quantum oscillation, he could nevertheless find nothing to suggest that you could not achieve a similar result to that provided by the £339.60 Bioshield by spending £5 on a USB key and putting a sticker on it.

I set about working out who was behind the device. A search in Companies House showed the directors of Bioshield Distribution included an Anna Grochowalska. She appeared to have been involved previously in a business called Immortalis, which sold a dietary supplement called Klotho Formula. Its website – rather similar in design to that for the Bioshield – said the product made use of a 'proprietary procedure that leads to relativistic time dilation and biological quantum entanglement at the DNA level'.

After I contacted Anna Grochowalska she came back insisting that while her company was the sole global distributor of the 5G Bioshield it did not manufacture or own the product. As for the science behind it: 'We are in possession of a great deal of technical information, with plenty of back-up historical research . . . As you can understand we are not authorized to fully disclose all this sensitive information to third parties for obvious reasons.' Aha: trade secrets, you see . . . She rejected any suggestion that selling a £5 product for more than £300 was unreasonable:

> In regard to the costs analysis your research has produced, I believe that the lack of in-depth information will not drive you to the exact computation of our expenses and production costs, including

the cost of IP rights, and so on. It is therefore hard to take your evaluation seriously, since you have evidently not researched the background facts in any meaningful way.

She wanted to put me in touch with the scientist behind the product, a Dr Lakicevic, but we decided the story was clear enough.

I asked Toby Hall why he found the device useful, and why he had thought it appropriate to recommend it in what was supposed to be a weighty official report on the science behind 5G. He replied that he had no regrets about buying the 5G Bioshield, and since plugging it in had felt beneficial effects. These had included being able to sleep through the night and having more dreams: 'I also felt a "calmer" feel to the home.'

But both Ken Munro and I had separately contacted London Trading Standards about this apparently worthless product for which unsubstantiated claims were being made. Its officers launched an investigation, and then sought a court order to have the Bioshield website taken down. 'We consider it to be a scam,' Stephen Knight, operations director for London Trading Standards, told me.

When this news broke, Glastonbury Town Council edited the full 5G report published on its website to remove the name of the device recommended by Toby Hall, with a note saying it had been redacted for legal purposes. It also released a sniffy statement alleging that my article about the device had failed to make it clear that the council had never recommended the product: it had simply been a 'member of the public'. Of course, that member of the public had been selected as someone with the expertise to help the council to understand 5G and the potential threat it posed.

A month or so later, there was a surprising postscript. A long email arrived from Toby Hall in which he told me that 'Your article has taken me on an extended journey of exploration.' At the end of it he had decided, lo and behold, that the device he had bought and recommended was in fact a scam. But there was a twist. 'The strange thing is the "scamsters" launched their scam off a genuine product made by Russian scientists that they had been promoting and selling.'

Oh, dear. He had convinced himself that an identical product to the 5G Bioshield called the Rezotone, which I had also seen being promoted by some of the flakier 5G conspiracy theorists, was in fact the genuine article. It was a somewhat depressing reminder that the battle between pseudoscience and the real thing is long and hard, and that people who believe in phoney scare stories and magical cures for imaginary conditions can rarely be convinced to change their minds.

I have dwelt at length on what happened in Glastonbury because it seems to tell a story about our love–hate relationship with the technology that has shaped our lives over the last decade or so. I have family who live not far from the town, and they have another complaint: getting a decent internet connection is a real struggle. Their mobile signal – just a couple of miles from the Glastonbury festival site where EE had experimented with 5G – is also very sketchy. The broadband company had offered to lay a fibre-optic cable up the country lane where they lived, but only if my relatives and their neighbours clubbed together to raise something like £30,000.

When I tried to video-call them during the coronavirus lockdown, we often had to give up, because the picture and sound kept freezing. Like other local people, my family did have some concerns about whether 5G was really safe. But in the pandemic, when their children were trying to do lessons online, or they were trying to run a craft business via Instagram and Facebook, the value of good connectivity became ever clearer.

The irony, of course, is that fast mobile internet connections and modern social networks don't just put a world of information and entertainment at our fingertips: they also flood us with a tidal wave of rumours, lies and hateful content. To be fair, social media sites have also helped scientists and fact-checkers to get their message across, but sometimes it feels as though the fake news is winning the online battle.

Throughout the pandemic the Oxford internet Institute produced a weekly report on misinformation about the virus distributed on social media. The researchers counted the number of articles about

COVID-19 from three sources: mainstream news, what it called 'junk health news', and a third category, 'state-backed news', which referred mainly to Russian and Chinese news sites. In one week in July 2020 the Institute painted what at first appeared to be a positive picture. Mainstream articles reached over 3 billion social media users, far outstripping the reach of state-backed and junk news. But when it looked at the levels of engagement for individual articles – how often they were retweeted, or liked on Facebook, or generated comments on Reddit – it was the state-backed and junk news sources that were well ahead of the mainstream media. Articles headlined '5G Is A Weapons System Designed To Kill' or 'Hydroxychloroquine – A Miracle Cure' seemed to be more engaging than ones explaining that 5G mast emissions had been found to be well within safe limits, or that the supposed wonder drug might have dangerous side-effects.

Looking at the impact of this constant stream of misinformation, at the way social networks appear to have magnified social and political divisions and threatened to undermine democracy, and at the addictive nature of the phones that have helped make all this possible, it would be easy to get depressed. The global health crisis was making us all dependent as never before on the technology of the social smartphone era. Tools which a few years earlier – during the Arab Spring or the London Olympics – had seemed life-enhancing, now appeared malign. But I am by nature an optimist, so let's end by pulling together some of the threads from this book and trying to weave a brighter picture of what technology could do for us.

EPILOGUE

As autumn arrived in 2020, I handed over the completed manuscript of this book to my publisher. But as the weather turned miserable and the rain lashed against the windows of the loft room where I had been writing, several issues right at the heart of *Always On*'s argument remained unresolved. In our journey between hope springing from the promise of what smartphones and social media could deliver and fear of the possibly malign consequences, the closing months of the year might, it came to seem to me, be crucial in determining whether we were heading into the light or the darkness.

Would Apple, which had signalled the arrival of the smartphone era when it unveiled the iPhone in 2007, propel the technology forward again by showing off a 5G iPhone? As a resurgence in the coronavirus made tracing those who might be infected even more urgent, would the National Health Service finally roll out a smartphone app that proved an effective addition to the government's armoury? And would the reputation of social media, already under fire as the superspreader of misinformation about the coronavirus, be further damaged as President Donald Trump and Joe Biden slugged it out in their race for the White House?

The answer to the first of these questions came quickly. Ever since that event in January 2007 at which it had launched the phone that went on to become the world's single most profitable product, September had been the month when Apple launched its latest iPhones. In recent years such occasions, with Tim Cook trying to whip up the same level of excitement in a whooping crowd as his predecessor Steve Jobs, had fallen a little flat. After all, each new rectangular slab of glass might well be 'the best iPhone we have ever made', but it looked much the same as the last.

In 2020, there was a different challenge. The coronavirus pandemic had meant delays in kitting out the Chinese factories making the new phone, and so the launch took place in October. What's more, it had to be a virtual event, without all those *ooohs*, *aaah*s and whoops from the onlookers in the hall.

Still, in an hour-long, slickly produced video presentation, Cook did his best to hammer home one key marketing message to his global online audience: *the iPhone is going 5G and that is a huge moment*. He tried to explain what this new high-speed network would mean: not just faster downloads and uploads, but 'higher-quality video streaming, more responsive gaming, real-time interactivity and so much more!' He brought the head of the US mobile operator Verizon on to his virtual stage to get even more excited about 5G and what it would signify for those who bought the new phone.

But both of them struggled to come up with compelling reasons why it would transform the experience of using a phone for people who were not playing high-concept video games on the train home. The real appeal of 5G is that it provides more capacity at pinch points on crowded networks, so that in future you might not see that spinning wheel of doom as you try to load a web page while passing through a mainline station. But that is a rather mundane message when you are trying to convince people they need to splash out £1,000 on another new phone.

As the presentation continued, the focus switched to something even more geeky: Apple's new A14 Bionic processor at the heart of the iPhone 12. This, to be fair, was a wonder of our modern world – the first 5nm (nanometre) chip. In other words, each transistor was just 25 atoms wide, meaning a total of 11.8 billion could be crammed in. Just to compare, back in 2007 a 90nm chip was in the first iPhone, and a chip expert tells me that means the 2020 version is roughly 64 to 70 times as powerful. Moore's Law, which said the number of transistors on a chip would double every two years, was no longer quite accurate, but its impact on the technology of the iPhone over 13 years was clear. The first phone was not even 3G, had a 2-megapixel camera with no video capability, and had maximum storage of 16GB.

It also only had a handful of apps, chosen by Apple. The 5G iPhone 12 Pro had a 12-megapixel camera with three lenses, could shoot 4K video good enough for a feature film, and had up to 512GB storage. And users could now choose from over 2 million apps. This device, just like the flagship phones from Apple's rivals Samsung and Huawei, was a stunning piece of technology, an illustration of just how far the smartphone revolution had come.

But whereas the original iPhone had seemed to me and millions of others a miraculous advance, my reaction to the latest model in October 2020 was, I suspect, similar to that of many people: 'Well, that's nice, but, whatever . . .' Just as in the television era we had become indifferent to the miracle of seeing live pictures beamed from as far away as the Moon, so it had taken us only a few years to accept as a given that we could carry with us tiny computers that could do everything from shoot a movie to respond to any question you could throw at them.

What was still not clear in the autumn of 2020, however, was whether the smartphone could help in the urgent task that preoccupied us all: controlling the spread of COVID-19. There was some good news about the NHS contact tracing app, which had been put on hold in June when it became apparent that the technology would not work without the co-operation of Google and Apple. A new version built using their privacy-focused framework was rolled out across England and Wales in late September; Scotland and Northern Ireland had already launched their own apps, using the same system.

The NHS COVID-19 app had a clever marketing ploy, in that it included a QR scanner, allowing you to check in at pubs, restaurants and other businesses without actually having to write down your phone number or email address. Quickly it became commonplace for just about every place you visited to have a code displayed in the window, a cue for people to download the app.

There were some initial teething troubles: the app would not work on older phones, and some people received phantom messages about exposure to the virus, which disappeared when you clicked on them. This latter problem caused plenty of confusion and was very poorly explained to the public. It appeared that the messages were being triggered automatically when the app asked the Apple or Google system for more information about the proximity between two phones to determine whether it crossed the threshold of a risky contact – one lasting 15 minutes at a distance of less than 2 metres. The Department of Health press office, under siege on all sorts of issues including the shambolic manual Test and Trace programme, seemed to have neither the knowledge nor the desire to explain anything about the workings of the app. It was only when I had a long chat with one of the technicians working on the app that I got even halfway to understanding what was going on. But overall it got a reasonable reception, with 19 million downloads in the first month. That was roughly the same as Germany's app, which was serving a population of 83 million, compared with the 57 million in England and Wales.

But was it working, ensuring that people who had been in contact with the virus were informed, so that the chain of infection was broken? That was just about impossible to know. As the developers of the German and Swiss apps had told me, the privacy built into the Apple and Google framework meant very little data came back to each country's health authority about how they were functioning. There was some information about how many positive tests had been entered into the app, and then how many alerts had been sent out warning people that they had been in contact with an infected person and needed to go into isolation. But what was not known, in Northern Ireland or Scotland or Germany, or indeed across England and Wales, was the identity of the people who had received the isolation alerts, and whether they had complied with their instructions. That led to a whole lot of head-scratching from civil servants at the launch of the NHS COVID-19 app when they were asked about the legal force of alerts sent out by the app. After all, if you got a phone call from the Test and Trace operation telling you to go into isolation, a failure to comply could lead to a fine of up to £10,000. Eventually they concluded that, as they could not know the identity of app users, complying with any alerts would have to be voluntary, although that also meant that people on low incomes could not apply for the £500 grant available to those ordered in a phone call to stay off work.

The consequences of the decisions taken over the spring and summer, under pressure from privacy campaigners, to guarantee that the app would know as little as possible about its users, were becoming apparent. Users who were probably totally unaware of that debate were asking some tricky questions. Why for instance, did an app which told you what the coronavirus alert level was in the area where you lived, not respond when you travelled to an area on higher alert? And why did some people get two different risk-level notifications for the area? The answer was that all the app knew about your location was the first half of your postcode, which you entered when you installed it. That could be a fairly wide area, and include districts with different risk levels – the developers had been told by the data regulators that if people entered their full postcode then it would be too easy to 'deanonymize' them.

They had also promised the public at an early stage that the app would not track their location, merely their phone's proximity to other phones with the NHS COVID-19 Bluetooth tracking switched on. That meant that it could not know when the user moved to a riskier neighbourhood, although if they scanned a QR code at a business later identified as a virus hotspot they might get an alert. Even then it would be couched in very general terms – 'Look out for any symptoms' – and would not identify the location where you might have been exposed to the virus.

Those who had lobbied for the NHS to follow the decentralized, privacy-focused Apple/Google approach had argued that it was the only way to get a wide cross-section of the public to trust the app and install it. Certainly, if you look at France's disaster with its centralized app – which even the Prime Minister did not download – that argument has some merit. But it is worth stopping to ponder for a moment whether we got the balance between privacy and efficacy right in deciding on the design of the app, and how that feeds into the wider debate about our attitudes to our health data.

One person involved, not in the NHS app but in one developed in another part of the UK, told me he thought there had been a tendency to base its design to suit the wishes of the minority for whom privacy is all-important. He explained that the public at large had a more nuanced view, especially if you explored the issues in detail.

> If you ask someone how important it is that their health data is kept private, then they'll say it is vital. But if you then explain that the consequence can be that there is a lengthy bureaucratic process before their GP can share their medical records with a hospital consultant, they'll say that's barmy.

This struck a chord with me. As someone who had spent some years being treated by the NHS for two serious conditions, I had been frustrated by how paper-based the bureaucracy had been, and how difficult it had proved to get different parts of the health service to share my data. The pandemic did at least seem to have led to some relaxation of rigid rules about data security: a friend treating seriously ill elderly patients told me that a previous reluctance to allow them to use phones or tablets to communicate with friends and relatives over the hospital's network had evaporated as the virus took hold.

An app, or technology more generally, was never going to be the answer to halting the coronavirus and saving hundreds of thousands of lives in the way it was described to me back in the spring. For that it became clear that an old-fashioned, smoothly functioning testing-and-tracing operation was needed. In the event, the NHS COVID-19 app made a small but useful contribution, and I encouraged everyone I knew to install it. But would a more intrusive attitude to data collection have been better, both in terms of controlling the virus and limiting the damage to the economy?

Look, for instance, at South Korea. In early March it had launched a smartphone app which tracked people sent into quarantine and alerted health officials if they left home without permission. That would have been completely unacceptable in the UK, but by late October South Korea had seen fewer than 500 deaths from the virus out of a population of 52 million. By then 45,000 people had died in the UK, and many millions of people were being forced back into lockdown, an arguably greater attack on their civil liberties than having their smartphones tracked. What is more, the Korean economy was beginning to emerge from recession, and looked certain to have suffered far less damage than the UK and many other countries were experiencing.

What was strange about the UK is that we seemed to trust our government with our secrets less than we trusted Apple and Google, which had been allowed to determine the shape of health policy, at least when it came to the app.

Meanwhile over in the United States, it seemed nobody trusted any institution – not the government, not the mainstream media, and certainly not the tech giants – as the most divisive election campaign in recent history rolled towards its conclusion.

As we have seen, Facebook's role in allowing Donald Trump's 2016 campaign to send millions of micro-targeted adverts crafted for individual voters had led to all kinds of inquests. Mark Zuckerberg, who initially laughed off what he deemed the 'crazy' idea that his company could have swung the election, was forced to eat humble pie. So in 2020 the spotlight was on Facebook and other social media platforms, amid a growing sense that they posed a real threat to democracy. This time around, it soon became clear that the danger was not so much the micro-targeting of voters but a tidal wave of misinformation shared across the platforms, not just in adverts but in posts by users. It ranged from the QAnon conspiracy theory, which painted President Trump as leading a fight against a satanic paedophile cult, to misinformation about when and how to vote. Fake rumours about the two presidential candidates abounded: Joe Biden was wearing an earpiece feeding him the answers in a debate, Donald Trump had an oxygen supply tube under his jacket when he emerged from hospital after being treated for coronavirus.

This time, Facebook and the other social media firms were eager to show they were aware of their influence and would do whatever it took to make sure their platforms were not abused. In Twitter's case that meant an outright ban on political advertising, but Facebook decided not to go that far. It would allow the campaigns to advertise, and would not police them for misinformation unless that related to the process of voting itself.

Soon that policy was under pressure, though, as the political temperature rose and the sheer volume of misinformation threatened to swamp the company's defences. In late September I joined other journalists on a call with Nick Clegg, the former UK Deputy Prime Minister who was now Facebook's global PR supremo. He wanted to tell us that things would not go wrong this time around: 'The company has changed a great deal since the 2016 US election. We're better prepared than ever before: we're working around the clock to protect the election from people who want to abuse our platforms, interfere or sow confusion.'

But it felt to me as though Facebook was continually having to adjust its policies to deal with new threats to the election. It had just announced that there would be a halt to any new political ads a week before polling day. I asked Clegg whether there were circumstances in which they might press the stop button earlier if the flow of misinformation became too much.

That wasn't going to happen, he insisted, because of all the safeguards they had put in place. He went on to defend political ads on Facebook as being no different from TV, radio and print ads – 'quite simply the lifeblood of democracy'.

Facebook did not call an early halt to those ads, but did have to keep adjusting its policies. In August it had begun removing some QAnon accounts that promoted violence; the day after the Clegg conference call it announced that it was going to stop people from running ads supporting the movement; finally, a week later, it banned any Facebook or Instagram accounts, groups or pages connected to the conspiracy theory.

But it was too late. By then the bizarre and dangerous movement which had been born three years earlier had gone mainstream, with even President Trump signalling his tacit approval when asked to condemn it on television. Even in the UK, a poll conducted by the anti-racism organization Hope Not Hate found that 6 per cent of those questioned said they supported QAnon, and 25 per cent agreed that 'secret Satanic cults exist and include influential elites'. That this poisonous ideology infected millions in the United States and beyond can only have been because its ideas were shared widely on the world's most powerful media platform.

Meanwhile, as Facebook and other social media firms tried belatedly to take action on this and other examples of misinformation, they found themselves in conflict with both the President and the wider Republican movement. Just six days before the election, the chief executives of Facebook, Twitter and Google were summoned to appear before Congress. The subject at issue was Section 230, the law framed in 1996 which essentially gave internet companies protection from lawsuits over what their users posted on their services.

But it was largely an opportunity for Republican senators to berate Mark Zuckerberg (Facebook), Jack Dorsey (Twitter) and Sundar Pichai (Google) over what they perceived as the anti-conservative bias of their platforms. Democrats, meanwhile, lambasted them for not going far enough in dealing with abusive behaviour. It was a bruising three-hour session which did not bode well for future relations between the tech giants and politicians from either side.

Election Day arrived on 3 November and, soon after the polls closed, it became clear that the social media firms were facing their biggest challenge yet. While the race was much tighter than the opinion polls had suggested, Joe Biden was heading inexorably towards victory. But in the White House Donald Trump was having none of it, sending out a stream of tweets and Facebook posts claiming he had won and the Democrats were trying to steal the election from him by fraudulent means. For once, Twitter and Facebook acted swiftly, plastering the President's posts with warning messages – 'This claim about election fraud is disputed' or 'Joe Biden is the projected winner of the 2020 US presidential election.'

But as the President and other Republicans whipped up their voters into a frenzy of anger over the 'stolen' election, Facebook in particular struggled to cope with the sheer volume of information on its platform. The Biden camp thought it was failing to live up to its promise to protect the democratic process: 'If you thought disinformation on Facebook was a problem during our election, just wait until you see how it is shredding the fabric of our democracy in the days after,' tweeted the President-elect's spokesman Bill Russo, before describing how right-wing sources were flooding the site with falsehoods. Former Obama speechwriter Ben Rhodes had even stronger language. 'It will take a generation to undo the damage that Facebook has done to American democracy and discourse,' he said. And, he warned, 'the fact that the leading source of information in America is a profit algorithm-driven cesspool of disinformation and hate speech has to be addressed through regulation.'

But the election result did not change perceptions of *any* of the tech giants for the better. Google still faced a landmark anti-trust lawsuit, launched by the Trump administration, over the way it maintained its dominance in search. Apple was under the spotlight over its treatment of its developers, Amazon over the power it had to determine which goods made it into our homes. And as for Facebook, it wasn't just politicians and regulators who had turned against it: even many of its billions of users now seemed convinced that it had made life worse, not better.

So how do I see the balance sheet of good and ill for this social smartphone era? Over the last decade I too had been on that journey of hope and fear. I was enthralled by many of the gadgets I encountered – the iPhone, the Raspberry Pi, the Amazon Echo – not only because they delivered real benefits to me in making both work and play more pleasurable, but also because they appeared to show that technology was being democratized.

This time the revolution was distributing these innovative tools more widely than ever before. Hardly anyone got to fly on Concorde, and while the domestic devices of the post-war era – washing machines, dishwashers, vacuum cleaners – were liberating for many, they were not as widely available as smartphones became in the twenty-first century. On a visit to Kenya I came across people who did not have running water or mains power, but owned phones which allowed them to use the Mpesa system to send money to relatives.

Once my phone was coupled with social media networks, I found it enriched my life, giving me a connection to people I would never have met otherwise. In particular, talking about both Parkinson's and my treatment for a malignant melanoma put me in touch with all sorts of people who wanted to share their experiences of the two conditions. In 2019, I spent a week having proton beam therapy on my eye at a hospital on the Wirral. I shot and edited a video diary about my experience with my phone and posted it online, something that would have been nigh-on impossible a decade earlier. On three or four occasions since then, people who are about to undergo the same treatment for this very rare condition have contacted me, having seen the video. I have been able to give them some reassurance.

But of course there is a very dark side to this revolution which has given millions the freedom to reach out around the world and express themselves for good or ill. That is perhaps best expressed by Leonard Pozner, whose son was among the schoolchildren killed in the Sandy Hook massacre in Connecticut in 2012, and who was then tormented by conspiracy theorists who said it had never happened. 'History books will refer to this period as a time of mass delusion,' he told the *Guardian* in 2017. 'We weren't prepared for the internet. We thought the internet would bring all these wonderful things, such as research, medicine, science, an accelerated society of good. But all we did was hold up a mirror to society, and we saw how angry, sick and hateful humans can be.'

Why, then, do I retain my optimism? While Leonard Pozner is right to say that we were deluded in our utopianism about the promise of the technology, we have at least woken from our dream. A new generation that has grown up with smartphones is more savvy about both their potential for creativity and their dangers, often proving more cautious than older people about how much they share online. Meanwhile clever people, from Tim Berners-Lee to Martha Lane Fox and Jimmy Wales, are coming up with ways to make the Web and social media function better for everyone and give us more control over our data.

There is also now a growing consensus that we need to regulate the tech giants, not just to make them protect people from abuse and hatred online, but to allow the next wave of innovators to challenge them and perhaps topple them from their perches. And those innovators could bring us all manner of wonders over the next decade. Having grown ever larger, the smartphone may shrink again, disappearing into new formats. Perhaps smart glasses better executed than the clunky Google Glass, or even contact lenses with screens activated by a voice command when you need them, will deliver us a less obtrusive 'always on' connection.

Artificial intelligence will be at the heart of the next wave of innovation and, while it will continue to be overhyped, it should start delivering real benefits. These will range from speeding up the process of discovering new drugs to helping us battle climate change by teaching our homes, our cars and the data centres on which society now runs to be more energy-efficient. The automation that AI brings has been seen as a threat to jobs, but so far the evidence shows that it is often augmenting humans rather than replacing them, helping radiologists process far more scans, for example, or taking the drudgery out of writing software and making it a more creative process.

Artificial intelligence has its dangers, with algorithmic bias a more immediate threat than killer robots destroying mankind, but this time we are better prepared. It was only after smartphones and social media were well established that we began to worry about the consequences, but already there appear to be almost as many researchers looking into the ethics of AI as there are trying to develop new applications for it.

Every invention has at first seemed a threat to the way we live. The spinning jenny took skilled work out of the home and into the factory. The internal combustion engine put the horse-and-carriage trade out of business and later polluted our cities. Television seemed to mean the end of cinema – and of family fun around the piano. But just as we cannot return to some pre-industrial age, so we cannot uninvent the iPhone or Facebook, nor should we want to. For millions of people the possession of a smartphone and the ability to connect to others via a social network has been transformational. For some it has enabled them to get educated, start their own business or learn vital information about their health. For others, particularly over the last year, it has provided an essential way of keeping in contact with loved ones at a time of loneliness and fear. The social smartphone era has only just begun. There is still time to shape these twenty-first-century tools so that they can be a boon, not a burden, for humanity.

ACKNOWLEDGEMENTS

This book was born out of a number of conversations with Jamie Birkett of Bloomsbury who encouraged me to take stock of my years covering the technology revolution and draw some lessons from it, something this news reporter driven by constant deadlines often fails to do. Throughout the process he has been a wise and calming presence, guiding me back on to the straight and narrow path whenever I got distracted or discouraged.

My agent Elly James has been a wonderful sounding board, full of encouragement when I needed it most. Thanks also to my copyeditor Graham Coster, who made many useful suggestions to improve my prose and tighten up key sections of the narrative. Ben Wood, with his unrivalled knowledge of the mobile phone industry, and Wikipedian and cryptocurrency specialist David Gerard each read sections of the book and gave me valuable advice about their specialist subjects.

Any number of colleagues at the BBC also deserve thanks. I joined the corporation as a researcher on Look North in Leeds in 1981 and have gone on to spend my whole career there. Broadcasting is a business replete with strong egos, but you quickly discover that it is also a team game. In writing this book, I have been reminded once again that the work I have done as a technology journalist would not have been possible without the help of dozens of talented and dedicated people who usually get little credit for what appears on air.

Camera operators, video editors and broadcast engineers too numerous to mention have saved my bacon over the years – and nowadays people like Steve Adrain do all of these jobs at once.

Producers have shaped my scripts, fixed up interviews with people I said would definitely not want to talk, and achieved the impossible by turning concepts such as quantum computing into watchable television. Jat Gill, Priya Patel, Carolyn Rice, Lakhvir Gill and

Jonathan Sumberg are just a few who have helped me and tolerated my terrible driving and lack of sangfroid in an edit suite as a deadline approaches.

In recent years I've worked ever more closely with the BBC's small but extraordinarily effective online technology news team, led by the indefatigable Leo Kelion. He and Jane Wakefield, Zoe Kleinman, Chris Fox, Dave Molloy – and, until he was wisely snapped up by the *FT*, Dave Lee – are brilliant journalists with deep knowledge of their subject and they have been an inspiration.

But my greatest debt is to my wife Diane Coyle. Over the last twenty years she has managed to write a whole series of brilliant books, many dealing with the economics of technology, without making any fuss. My writing process has been a whole lot noisier and more disruptive to the household but throughout Diane has been extraordinarily patient, offering sympathy, sound advice about subjects such as technology's productivity paradox, and endless cups of tea. She signed up to 'in sickness and in health' but putting up with a husband writing a book during a pandemic was never mentioned. Thank you, Diane.

INDEX